Endorse

- **Rev. Richard Rohr, O.F.M.** — "At the very least, we should be able to presume that the Gospel creates healthy and happy people, especially among those who speak in God's name. Yet we know this is not the norm and even the opposite is often the case. Nicholas Amato describes what is often the heart of the problem and shows us the way through and forward."
  ❧ Center for Action and Contemplation, Albuquerque, New Mexico

- **Rev. James Martin, S.J.** — "Msgr. Nicholas Amato's second book guides those in ministry and others from stress to joy. His spiritual mastery honed over nearly five decades of priesthood encourages the reader to seek God's voice within; to find God in all; and, to build bridges in all seasons despite set-backs or failure. Like Simone Weil in her *Notebooks*, he grasps that 'waiting patiently, in expectation, is the foundation of the spiritual life.' He embraces joy, humor and laughter as constitutive elements of spiritual growth. Msgr. Amato emerges as a true spiritual father whose contemplative bent and rich pastoral history yield a vision gentle in manner and resolute in approach."
  ❧ Editor-at-Large, *America Magazine*, author, *Jesus: A Pilgrimage*

- **Rev. Stan Gumula, O.C.S.O.** — "The second Abbot of Mepkin, Father Christian Aidan Carr, was fond of saying: 'Where there is more truth, there is more joy.' What better words could be found to describe Father Amato's newest book? Wedding psychology and contemplative prayer can bring us into the realms of both more truth and more joy. As an Associate of Mepkin Abbey, he has opened us monks to the joy which resides at the deepest levels of our hearts, a joy which is only released when we bring our daily lives with all its pains before the loving presence of the One God."
  ❧ Abbot of Mepkin Abbey

- **Dr. Robert McAllister** — "This isn't just a book; it's a two year course in contemplative prayer. It's a very thorough and erudite discussion and explanation of prayer life."
  ❧ Retired Psychiatrist, Professor, Author

- **Mr. Rich Lewis** — "Do you want to reclaim the inner joy that God has planted within you? Pleasure is in the body; happiness is in the mind, but joy is a deeper reality at the center of who we are. God unconditionally loves us and wishes that we will discover this inner joy that bubbles below the surface of our lives. Nicholas shares practical tools that will help us identify and manage our daily experience of stress so we can more easily move into contemplative prayer and reclaim God's gracious gift of inner joy."
  ❧ Author and founder of *www.SilenceTeaches.com*

- **Rev. Gerald S. Twomey** — "Like his earlier book, *Living in God: Contemplative Prayer and Contemplative Action*, Monsignor Nicholas Amato's latest offering, *Moving from Stress to Joy*, rewards the reader with a feast of reason and a flow of soul. Amato's four decades of parish ministry, retreat work, parish missions, spiritual direction and counseling result in this warm and inviting book, reminiscent of such spiritual guides as Morton Kelsey, Henri J.M. Nouwen, Anthony deMello, S.J., Joan Chittister, O.S.B., John Sanford, Rose Mary Dougherty, Gerald May, M.D., Thomas Keating, O.C.S.O. and James Martin, S.J. Amato writes with a flair, popular in the best sense. He invests his work with insights and awareness born from the experience of a pastor 'who knows the smell of the sheep.' His close contemplative ties with a Trappist monastery and long-time staff affiliation with a clinical psychiatric center yield rich insights, awareness and applications. In this stress-filled era, like Pierre Teilhard de Chardin, S.J. Amato reminds us: 'Joy is the infallible sign of the presence of God.'"
  ❧ Editor. *Thomas Merton: Prophet in the Belly of a Paradox* (Paulist Press), *Remembering Henri: The Life and Times of Henri J.M. Nouwen* (Orbis Books)

- **Sr. Mary Therese White, O.S.F.** — "Father Nicholas has written a well-researched look at the reality of stress in the lives of modern people, as well as reflection on contemplative presence as a way to hold stress and go deeper to a place of true joy. He offers a practical approach to developing contemplative prayer, as well as practicing contemplative experience as awareness of God's joy-producing Presence in the midst of daily life."
  ❧ Former Provincial, Franciscan Sisters of Baltimore

- **Sr. Patricia Kirk, O.S.B.** — "*Moving from Stress to Joy* is a book I have been waiting for, (even without naming) for quite a while. Seeing the words stress and joy together is comforting knowing that God is in the midst of both. Contemplative presence and stress reduction are tangible tools - gifts from God. God is not only in the joy but as we open ourselves and take the necessary steps will lead us beyond the stress. As Fr. Amato, reminds us "we were created out of joy!" We need to claim that gift."
  ❧ Prioress of Emmanuel Monastery in Baltimore, MD

Moving from Stress to Joy

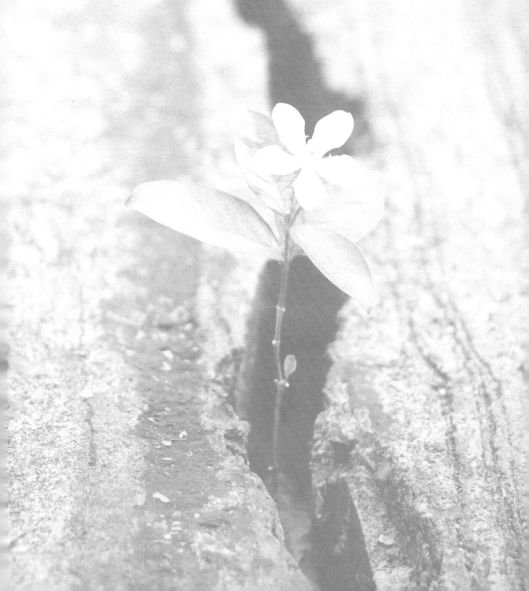

Moving from Stress to Joy

NICHOLAS AMATO

UPTOWN PRESS, INC.
Baltimore, Maryland
2018

Layout & Design by: Uptown Press, Inc.
                            Baltimore, MD
                            www.uptownpress.com

ISBN: 978-1-935911-22-7

To my parents, Mary and Paul, who always seemed able to label and name their stress in the moment, and more importantly, for the ways they taught us children, through their actions, to reclaim the inner joy of being alive, belonging to a family, and being loved by God.

Contents

Acknowledgements

There are many who have contributed to my writing of this book, but it is to my readers who offered their professional experience and expertise in its careful editing. I am indebted to Ed Arsenault, the former President and CEO of St. Luke Institute, both as a psychiatrist and spiritual director; Father Paul Byrnes for his expertise as a pastoral care minister; Reverend Greg Cochran for his gifts of spiritual direction as a Baptist minister; Ms. Jane Deaton as a lay woman committed to contemplative prayer; Ms. Beth Taneyhill, who has served many years as a parish Faith Formation Director; Ms. Maureen Yantz, as a woman committed to daily prayer and volunteering and ministering in her local parish; and Cindi Stewart, who deserves heartfelt thanks for editing the final draft.

Foreword

What is it like living in our world today? For most of us I expect we would include words like "fast paced;" "constantly changing;" "demanding yet valued family and work life;" "over-loaded with internet and other sources of information, opinion, entertainment, and relationships;" "confronting sometimes conflicting religious, cultural, ethnic and political values and groups; wanting to find safety and peace in a country armed with over 300,000 civilian guns hidden in jackets and closets, and suffering many unpredictable acts of violence;" "wanting to discern what is ours to do that can contribute to the ever-evolving common good;" "finding a few islands of slow living in our lives, where we can smell the flowers and just appreciate what's given in the moment." We could go on and on. It's an exhaustingly exciting and sometimes depressing time in which to live.

Where does such a world leave us? One answer is, enormously stressed. Another answer is, in the face of that debilitating stress a desire to find a way out of it. If we're spiritually alive we also desire to find ways that our faith practices can ground us and its scriptural promise of joy can be realized.

Nicholas Amato has given us inspired and extensive, very practical help in this book for: 1) understanding and managing our physical and psychological stress; 2) moving through and beyond it to a practice of contemplative prayer, where we let go the stressed ego level of our identity and dispose ourselves to realizing our true personal identity and freedom in God's love; 3) letting that love overflow through us into our hurting world; and finally 4) opening to the profound joy that grace raises up in us. I found it to be a hopeful book, raising up practical possibilities for moving toward a better life that we may have given up trying to find.

Father Amato brings his own extensive psychological, theological, pastoral and contemplative learning as well as many concrete personal experiences to bear in his writing. He also includes many deep insights from scripture and a wide range of religious writers, poets and other artists, stress specialists, and neuroscientists.

I think this book is a unique, wise contribution to all of us who want concrete help in reducing and managing the many forms of destructive physical and psychological stress we endure in our time, and who also want stress reduction to connect with the life of the spirit, especially through contemplative prayer and its way of leading us to a deeper, freer, compassionate sense of identity in God, and to the powerful gift of true joy. He carefully weaves all these dimensions together into a way to sane wholeness in our lives.

Rev. Tilden Edwards
Founder & Senior Fellow,
Shalem Institute for Spiritual Formation

A Note From the Author

This book arose out of years of leading retreats, parish missions, and days of recollection. Their contents included: learning about Centering Prayer, transforming prayer into effective action, dealing with stress, experiencing God's presence in our lives as Trinity, living a more compassionate life, living with monotony and difficult people, and growing in age and grace. I began to see how all of them were in several ways related as God's work in us, and out of this insight, I was encouraged to put my notes, exercises, and feedback from hundreds of retreatants into a book format. This is what I have attempted to do in the present work.

Having said that, I would like to share how this book could be used individually or with small groups for additional impact. To begin with, the chapters are sequential and developmental, that is, each can stand alone, yet each builds on the chapter that preceded it. Each of the chapters concludes with a set of questions with space to jot your reflections. If a small group is reading the book together, you might assign a chapter for each session — taking two sessions on the longer chapters — and when coming together, share any insight you may have had regarding the material, as well as your responses to each of the questions. This format was used with a contemplative aging reading group I belong to, and we have found it very useful. Individual appendices could also serve as a focus for a session, discussing for example in Appendix I which of the 45 Fruits of Contemplation you have seen come to pass in your own life, or which you would like to see and how your contemplative practice might contribute to achieving them. Finally, there is a worksheet in Appendix J. The worksheet could be useful as part of a Day in the Desert alone, or as part of a Day of Recollection spent with a small group. It includes directions for its use and uses the book as a starting point from which to gain a greater understanding in the steps for your own personal spiritual growth. In the aforementioned, we are following an experiential learning model rather than the old lecture method of the schools of our youth or even of many formats of retreats today. The experiential method aims at marrying information to personal experience and then articulating it for longer lasting impact and effect both on the individual and on others. Thus, you may readily see that my suggestions for working with the book include reading the material, experiencing the material using reflection questions at the end of the chapter, and then either sharing the reflections or journaling on them. The time spent on a monthly reprise serves as a checkpoint to see where you have been, where you are now, and where you might want to move in the coming months. The quality of your prayer will change. Handling stress will indeed be improved. Joy and compassion will flow more easily.

The amount of stress with which we live, coupled with the lack of joy people experience, is the topic of this book. Both stress and joy need to be considered together, for while stress is the state in which most of us live, joy is the ultimate nature of reality. It grounds every created thing in the love the creator has for what has been created. Stress has a way of accumulating on us, like soot or oxidation on a valuable brass vase, masking the luster of the individual. Manage the stress, reconnect with the creator, and the vase begins to shine brilliantly to the joy of all who encounter it. We turn now to our first chapter where we will ground our considerations in contemporary psychology and spirituality.

Chapter 1: Introduction

Scriptural Grounding
1. A Deeper Meaning of the Annunciation
2. This Author's Experience

The Present Work
3. Why I Have Written this Book
4. What Will We Consider and How Will We Go About It?

A Work of Psychology and Spirituality
5. Grace and Nature; Nature and Grace
6. Psychology & Spirituality — the Best of Both Worlds
7. Can There Be a Psychology of Prayer?

A DEEPER MEANING
OF THE ANNUNCIATION

The reality hit her like a bolt of lightning, as if she'd never seen the impending clouds gathering off in the distance. In a moment, in the present... the sky split open, and the gaping reality before her rose in her heart; she was pregnant, and she couldn't imagine how this could have happened! She thought for sure she was, "a different type of girl!" In the course of what seemed like a few minutes, she could feel herself moving from consternation, confusion, and conflict through a quieting down, a gaining of an inner peace, and a movement to a moment of simple joy.

We are all familiar with the story, but it is the process of moving from stress to joy to which I would like to call our attention. Let us see what can be gleaned from the account made familiar by St. Luke.

> "In the sixth month of Elizabeth's pregnancy, God sent the angel Gabriel to Nazareth, a town in Galilee, to a virgin pledged to be married to a man named Joseph, a descendant of David. The virgin's name was Mary. The angel went to her and said, 'Greetings[1], you who are highly favored! The Lord is with you.'
>
> Mary was greatly troubled at his words and wondered what kind of greeting this might be. But the angel said to her, 'Do not be afraid, Mary; you have found favor with God. You will conceive and give birth to a son, and you are to call him Jesus. He will be great and will be called the Son of the Most High. The Lord God will give him the throne of his father David, and he will reign over Jacob's descendants forever; his kingdom will never end.'
>
> 'How will this be,' Mary asked the angel, 'since I am a virgin?'
>
> The angel answered, 'The Holy Spirit will come on you, and the power of the Most High will overshadow you. So the holy one to be born will be called the Son of God. Even Elizabeth your relative is going to have a child in her old age, and she who was said to be unable to conceive is in her sixth month. For no word from God will ever fail.'
>
> 'I am the Lord's servant,' Mary answered. 'May your word to me be fulfilled.' Then the angel left her."[2]

---

[1] The Greek word translated here as "Greetings" is *Xaire* which means "rejoice" as in the Jerusalem Bible Translation.

[2] Luke 1: 26–38 (New International Version).

Mary is clearly fearful and stressed over what will happen to her in the society of her day where women, pregnant out of wedlock, were subject to ridicule, ostracizing, and even death by stoning. She does, however, in the midst of her stress, receive a sense of consolation. Notice that she receives it with an open heart. When she questions, she is given assurance that she has found favor with God, no matter what the situation seems to be. An explanation, seemingly preposterous, is given to her regarding "next steps." She will be "overshadowed" by a Presence, and out of that Presence a son will be born to her. Still a bit incredulous, the assurance and the Presence are enough for her to hold the stress in a different way, that is to say, not to hold the stress at all, but to let it go. Note, it isn't an irresponsible or reckless letting go, but one of holding on to the assurance with one hand and letting go with the other. Once she is able to move through this simple process or paradigm, a sense of relief, inner peace, and joy flood her, out of which she speaks those beautiful words of response: "May your word to me be fulfilled." While the promise is still not fulfilled, it had become clear that she is now willing to cooperate with it and cooperate with it fully.

THIS AUTHOR'S EXPERIENCE

What I am able to relate to quite easily in Luke's account of the Annunciation are the many times I feel stressed, either from my own fears or imperfections, or from my ruminations about meeting a deadline, or having too much on my plate on a given day, or the stress arising from relationships. In those moments, what do I do, or what is available to me as a stress reducer? To answer these questions, I have gone to times when my stress moves through some sort of process to joy. I then go back and see what I did to facilitate the transition.

A few examples might serve us well here. For starters, there's the stress of having too much to accomplish in a given day. As the hours pass, the stress mounts until I am nervously pacing about. At such times, I find it helpful to acknowledge both my negative and positive emotions, to simply breathe deeply, and to break the whole up into smaller parts. The breathing brings me some calm. I will also include a word or two to focus on that relates to God's presence and compassion with and for me, such as "Be my light" or "Stand by me." The psychological and the spiritual components do put me in a better place. Without having lifted a finger, they physically change the situation.

Another example, perhaps more extreme, is not regularly saving sections of the manuscript as I am writing this book. Suddenly the computer freezes, and I lose the entire section. I cannot believe it is gone! Gone forever and not able to be reclaimed! Here, the stress and disillusionment hits me full force. I find myself wanting to cry out or act impetuously. Spontaneously and instantaneously, alternatives race through my mind: "Yes, I'll just eat myself to death!" or, "I'll rant and rave for a while." The psychological part of the transitioning will find me talking to myself: "It's not the end of the world!" "I will get through this." "Don't do anything rash." Over and over, I'll mention these or similar phrases. I am then able to breathe, sit in silence, and surface a word or very short phrase to take into a few moments of silence within. They might include: "Save me Lord." "Light in darkness." "I'm drowning."

In both these examples, the psychological situation is acknowledged, and the world of spirit is accessed. It is very similar to the situation in the Annunciation. Mary acknowledges her stress. She opens her heart and is calmed and able to receive a sense of consolation. Calming herself allows her to surrender to the wonderful and beautiful mystery that is God. The assurance from beyond confirms that she has found favor with God — no matter what the situation seems to be. Next steps for her to follow are then received. Such surrender is an example of what is known as *Apophatic theology*,[3] where my faith becomes the freedom not to know or understand something fully because I experience myself as being known more fully than I can ever know.[4] It is also affirmed in Paul's First Letter to the Corinthians where he states, "Now I know in part; then I shall understand fully, even as I have been fully understood."[5]

WHY I HAVE WRITTEN THIS BOOK

In reviewing the resources available in print and on the Internet, it becomes evident that much has been written on stress reduction. As a separate field of endeavor, lots has also been written on prayer as a way to experience inner peace. Two areas that have stirred me to write this book are how stress reduction from a psychological perspective might be wedded to prayer from a spiritual perspective so the transformation from stress to joy can be seen as a holistic experience. Second, how might contemplative prayer, in contrast to verbal/vocal prayer or meditation, be a resource in furthering this "marriage" of nature and grace? There is no reason why prayer — especially contemplative prayer — and stress need to be seen as two unrelated and separate disciplines. Even with that being said, I have found that in cases where their interrelatedness is acknowledged, it is verbal/vocal prayer or meditation that is considered. Rarely is contemplative prayer the element in the comparison.

---

[3] "The Mystica," accessed December 5, 2016, https://www.themystica.org.
[4] Richard Rohr, "Experience: Weekly Summary," Richard Rohr's Daily Meditation, January 28, 2017, accessed January 28, 2017, https://cac.org/experience-weekly-summary-2017-01-28/.
[5] 1 Corinthians 13:12, (Revised Standard Version).

WHAT WILL WE CONSIDER AND HOW WILL WE GO ABOUT IT?

I begin by asking two questions: "Are you under a great deal of stress?" "Have you tried pausing and turning to a way of praying that offers concrete and lasting results?" What I would like to offer the reader in this book is a practical way of determining his stress level and then acquiring a level of contemplative presence that opens him to an experience of deep joy. By the book's end, the reader will have gained practical tools for moving from a daily experience of the stresses associated with family, career, relationships, or senior living, to moments of reclaimed joy. With practice the use of these tools could become a new way of living out each day. Regular practice of the two techniques together could provide the possible formation of a routine that could become a life-enriching habit.

GRACE AND NATURE; NATURE AND GRACE

St. Thomas Aquinas, the great medieval Dominican theologian, taught that grace builds on nature. *The Catechism of the Catholic Church* summarizes well the interaction of God's grace and our human nature. The following is a summary of the passage numbers in this regard.[6]

> ➤ 1996: Our justification comes from the grace of God. Grace is favor, the free and undeserved help that God gives us to respond to his call to become children of God, adoptive sons, partakers of the divine nature and of eternal life.

> ➤ 1997: Grace is a participation in the life of God. It introduces us into the intimacy of Trinitarian life...

> ➤ 1998: This vocation to eternal life is supernatural. It depends entirely on God's gratuitous initiative, for he alone can reveal and give himself. It surpasses the power of human intellect and will, as that of every other creature.

> ➤ 1999: The grace of Christ is the gratuitous gift that God makes to us of his own life, infused by the Holy Spirit into our soul to heal it of sin and to sanctify it...

---

[6] *The Catechism of the Catholic Church*, 1996–1999, 2001–2003.

- ➢ 2001: The preparation of man [sic] for the reception of grace is already a work of grace. This latter is needed to arouse and sustain our collaboration in justification through faith, and in sanctification through charity. God brings to completion in us what he has begun…

- ➢ 2002: God's free initiative demands man's [sic] free response, for God has created man in his image by conferring on him, along with freedom, the power to know him and love him. The soul only enters freely into the communion of love. God immediately touches and directly moves the heart of man. He has placed in man a longing for truth and goodness that only he can satisfy.

- ➢ 2003: Grace is, first and foremost, the gift of the Spirit who justifies and sanctifies us. But grace also includes the gifts that the Spirit grants us to associate us with his work…

All creation becomes a virtual theater of God's grace and God's action made manifest. All creation, and our own human nature are, so to speak, a stage on which the drama of fuller life in God is coming to completion. Unlike later Protestant reformers that saw nature as evil and unredeemed, Thomas taught that God's grace, God's life, does not negate anything in the created world. To the contrary, grace builds up, renews, and completes the nature that is given. So, the stressed, anxious, overworked, and overextended individual can, through God's grace, not only be restored to former peace, but can be made new in a transformed way. Scriptures make it clear that this remarkable change is actually from within and by God's grace. The Psalms attest that we are "washed brighter than snow."[7] (Psalm 51:7) The secret may lie in acknowledging the stress and disposing us to the grace that transforms from within. The longing for this wholeness is very real, even though the reality may not yet be experienced. It is stronger than the fears or stresses we may be experiencing. Thomas states that, "Our preoccupation may be with avoiding the latter rather than seeking the former."[8] Only an honest admission and understanding of the stress can pave the way for taking it to prayer and having God work the transformation.

---

[7] Author's Note: The use of "brighter" rather than "whiter" goes easy on people of color.
[8] Summa Theologica, Ia-2ae xxxv, 6.

PSYCHOLOGY AND SPIRITUALITY, THE BEST OF BOTH WORLDS

In my almost 50 years of counseling individuals and couples, I have seen the changes that insight into one's behavior can achieve. When this process is brought to prayer, remarkable things can happen. Disposing yourself to God's presence and waiting upon the Lord, grace begins to flow. Reflection on your time in the presence starts to make a difference in your intentions and actions. This is the combining of nature and grace to achieve an enhanced benefit.

This combining became more explicit and real in the years I spent at St. Luke's Institute, a national behavioral rehabilitation center just outside of Washington, DC, for Catholic clergy and religious suffering with addictions and personality disorders. As one of five spiritual integrators on staff, I worked closely with the clinical staff in integrating the insights of therapy into the spiritual lives of the residents. It should be remembered that these folks had prayer lives, which they practiced with regularity since their formative days in novitiate or seminary. There was a common understanding among all staff that the first thing to go and the last thing to return was their prayer life. In the symbiotic role of nature and grace, it appears that as prayer (grace) decreases and ends, addictions and irregular behavior (nature) rise. While in the six-month residential program, initial efforts were made with regard to therapy (and thus address our *nature* as human beings), and over time, prayer and spirituality were reintroduced. Over each month, the interrelatedness of the two was increased and nature opened to grace and grace enhanced and sustained nature. By the time the individual was ready for discharge, old patterns of prayer had returned with fresh energy, or new ones had been formed. The experience of this interdependence often was expressed in small group sessions where residents would testify to a new sense of who they were apart from their compulsions, more explicitly, who they were in God. This book is not a substitute for intense psychotherapy or regular spiritual direction. It is, however, for someone who has tried verbal prayers or meditation as ways to deal with the stresses of family, friends, and workplace without much success. It is a resource available to anyone of any faith or religious tradition. It will offer the reader practices that uncover and clarify the stresses experienced in his life and assist him in uncovering the joy that lies within him.

CAN THERE BE A PSYCHOLOGY OF PRAYER?

My experience as a spiritual integrator has helped me see the powerful relationship of psychotherapy and spiritual direction, reaffirming the medieval understanding of nature's interaction with grace. It raises an additional question regarding a psychological perspective on prayer itself. One wonders whether there is a psychological underpinning to prayer. What does psychology have to say about it?

The husband and wife team of Ann and Barry Ulanov lectured and taught at Union Theological Seminary in New York City. She was a Jungian analyst who taught and wrote on religious thought and he, a professor of psychiatry and religion at the Seminary. In their joint work, *Primary Speech*,[9] they define prayer not only as God's reaching out to us, but as a coping tool that can assist someone in achieving a level of harmony in one's life. They wrote in an earlier work:

> "If we can let ourselves go in prayer and speak all that is in our minds and hearts, if we can sit quietly and bear the silence, we will hear all the bits and pieces of ourselves crowding in on us, pleading for our attention. Prayer's confession begins with this racket, for prayer is noisy with the clamor of all the parts of us demanding to be heard. The clamor is the sound of the great river of being flowing in us. This is what depth-psychologists call 'primary-process thinking,' that level of our psyche's functioning that leads straight to the workings of our souls."[10]

Almost every word in this quote opens us to the subject at hand: opening ourselves to prayer, sitting quietly, noting the "bits and pieces" of stress within us, being in touch with the yearning to be put at peace, and experiencing the "great river flowing beneath us." It is to this understanding of the harmony achieved between stress and joy to which this book is devoted.

---

[9] Ann and Barry Ulanov, *Primary Speech: A Psychology of Prayer,*
(Atlanta: John Knox Press, 1982).

[10] Ann and Barry Ulanov, *Religion and the Unconscious,* (Philadelphia: Westminster Press, 1975), 26–32.

Reflection Questions for Chapter 1: Introduction

❦ *In reading the description of the Annunciation in Chapter 1, what are your reactions to stress like?*

❦ *Select three stressful situations this past week and compare your reactions.*

❦ *What specific skills or techniques do you presently use to deal with each of the stressful situations?*

Chapter 2: Christian Joy

Joy
1. Joy Defined
2. Psychological and Spiritual Understanding of Joy
3. Joy in Sacred Scripture
4. Joy the Greatest of Gifts
5. Joy as a Secular Goal

Grace in Stillness
6. Mindfulness Strictly Defined
7. Joy, the Fruit of Contemplative Presence
8. Grace as Energy
9. Grace: The Power of Contemplative Presence

JOY DEFINED

To begin our consideration, it would serve us well to spend some time on our goal, namely to experience the emotion of joy. The dictionary defines joy as, "The emotion evoked by well-being, success, or good fortune or by the prospect of possessing what one desires." Secondarily, it adds "A state of happiness or felicity," and thirdly, "A source or cause of delight."[11] So joy is an emotion that arises from within by a stimulus that is perceived as important to the person. It may have the feel of delight, gaiety, or bliss.

PSYCHOLOGICAL & SPIRITUAL UNDERSTANDING OF JOY

C.S. Lewis captured the nuance between joy and pleasure well in his work, *Surprised by Joy* wherein he states:

> "As I stood beside a flowering currant bush on a summer day there suddenly arose in me without warning, and as if from a depth not of years but of centuries, the memory of that earlier morning at the Old House when my brother had brought his toy garden into the nursery. It is difficult to find words strong enough for the sensation which came over me…It was a sensation, of course, of desire; but desire for what?… Before I knew what I desired, the desire itself was gone, the whole glimpse…withdrawn, the world turned commonplace again, or only stirred by a longing for the longing that had just ceased… In a sense the central story of my life is about nothing else…The quality…is that of an unsatisfied desire which is itself more desirable than any other satisfaction. I call it Joy, which is here a technical term and must be sharply distinguished both from Happiness and Pleasure. Joy (in my sense) has indeed one characteristic, and one only, in common with them; the fact that anyone who has experienced it will want it again…I doubt whether anyone who has tasted it would ever, if both were in his power, exchange it for all the pleasures in the world. But then Joy is never in our power and Pleasure often is."[12]

---

[11] Merriam Webster Dictionary, s.v. "joy," accessed December 5, 2016, http://www.merriam-webster.com.

[12] C. S. Lewis, *Surprised by Joy: The Shape of My Early Life,* (Orlando: Harcourt, 1955), 18.

As Lewis says, the joy we crave is "never in our power" and "nothing can compare to it." We will soon see how true this is from the vantage point of sacred scripture, which speaks so beautifully of the world beyond, that can be touched in the individual through contemplative prayer.

While C.S. Lewis represents well the spiritual world, psychology today also speaks of joy from a more physiological or psychological perspective. There is today what is being called a *Psychology of Joy*. It is a multi-dimensional psychology that integrates philosophy, meditation, and unique creative processes, which support more mindful and loving states of consciousness. It should be noted that adherents speak of more secular, tangible, measurable means such as philosophy and meditation. These means aid in accomplishing a "Loving Space" in which all elements of the human psyche, the subconscious, conscious, and super conscious are integrated and from which personal transformation proceeds. "The purpose of Psychology of Joy is to provide unique understandings of human psychology and personal experiences that support individuals, families and communities to live profoundly joyous lives."[13]

Joy from a spiritual point of view then, is more than happiness, and happiness is more than pleasure. Pleasure is in the body. Happiness is in the mind and feelings, if you will, but joy is a deeper reality subsiding in the heart, the spirit, and the center of who we are. One spiritual writer holds that,

> "The way to pleasure is power and prudence. The way to happiness is moral goodness. The way to joy is sanctity, loving God with your whole heart and your neighbor as yourself. It is clear that everyone wants pleasure. More deeply, everyone wants happiness. Most deeply, everyone wants joy."[14]

From a psychological vantage point, joy is more the creating of a space of joy using human resources than it is the experiencing of something that whelms up from within.

JOY IN SACRED SCRIPTURE

Having distinguished between the psychological and spiritual aspects of joy, let us turn to the Psalms and words of Jesus regarding the reality in order to gain a more holistic understanding of the state that can be ours. The Psalms speak of joy in two ways, one being the inward experience and the second, a way of externally expressing that reality. We are more concerned with the former. Thus, I would cite the following Psalm passages to convey this inner experience.

---

[13] Jerry Rosser, "Psychology of Joy," Psychology of Joy, accessed December 5, 2016, http://www.psychologyofjoy.com.

[14] Peter Kreeft, "Joy," accessed December 5, 2016, http://www.peterkreeft.com/topics/joy.htm.

- ➤ Psalm 16:11 — "You make known to me the path of life; you will fill me with joy in your presence, with eternal pleasures at your right hand."

- ➤ Psalm 21:6 — "Surely you have granted him unending blessings and made him glad with the joy of your presence."

- ➤ Psalm 94:19 — "When anxiety was great within me, your consolation brought me joy."[15]

It should be noted that the joy experienced is a result of an inner presence to the speaker. That very presence is relational, that is, there is another "Being" who is present to the speaker. Secondly, this presence has an impact on the speaker of the Psalm, namely one of consolation. This will be an important consideration as we proceed, in the sense that we can have practices that calm us internally *and* enable us to relate to a Presence who will bring us a lasting and fully satisfying sense of peace and joy.

Let us turn for a moment to the Gospels for their own testimony to this inner experience of joy promised us in the Psalms. The Gospel of Matthew speaks of a seed falling on receptive ground where it is welcomed and received with joy and then takes root and flowers.[16] The earlier Gospel of Mark says the same.[17] The first two chapters of the Gospel of Luke are overflowing with joy; indeed the whole Gospel is colored by it. However, it is the 15th Chapter of John's Gospel that discloses the heart of the matter. In his Last Supper Discourse, knowing his end on this earth is near, Jesus shares truths with his followers. They are truths that will last them through thick and thin when he is absent.

> "As the Father has loved me, so have I loved you. Now remain in my love. If you keep my commands, you will remain in my love, just as I have kept my Father's commands and remain in his love. I have told you this so that my joy may be in you and that your joy may be complete."[18]

Joy "in" and joy "complete" speaks beautifully of this deeper spiritual, and very real presence that is relational between the individual follower and Jesus. He assures them that all they need to do is ask for this joy (John 16:24). He is telling them this now so they may have a full measure of the joy when he is gone.[19]

---

[15] Psalms 16:11, 21:6, 94:19, (Revised Standard Version).

[16] Matthew 13:1-9, (Revised Standard Version).

[17] Mark 4:1-9, (Revised Standard Version).

[18] John 15:9-11, 17, (Revised Standard Version).

[19] John 17:13, (Revised Standard Version).

JOY, THE GREATEST OF GIFTS

St. Thomas Aquinas affirms that, "No man [sic] can live without joy. That is why one deprived of spiritual joy goes over to carnal pleasures." Sanctity is never a substitute for sex, but sex is often a substitute for sanctity. Our experience assures us that Thomas is correct in his statement. No one who ever said to God, "Thy will be done" and meant it with his heart, ever failed to find joy in the present moment, much less have to await it in a future heaven. In the very act of self-surrender to God there can be joy, and not simply as a consequence, but in the very moment as we shall see. The symbolism and analogy to sexual surrender, say in the marriage relationship, holds for a man's soul as well as it does for a woman's. Peter Kreeft states that, "Only when lovers give up all control and melt helplessly into each other's bodies and spirits, only when they overcome the fear that demands control, do they find the deepest joy. Frigidity, whether sexual or spiritual, comes from egotism."[20] Surrender in contemplative prayer will be such a situation.

In our own lives, we can attest to the fact that so many people are stressed beyond levels of tolerance. Many acquire a survivor mentality because they simply have to get through the day, the week, the year. To do so, they will simply "gut it out," just hang on and not even acknowledge the level of stress they are experiencing, which soon is experienced as "normal." Eventually, the unacknowledged stress becomes the set-point and begins to feel like what normal should be. Their blood pressure, aches and pains, sleepless nights, nevertheless, will testify to another reality. The key will be how to move through the stress to the inherent joy that is bubbling just below the surface of their lives. Acknowledging stress, using natural practices to calm its turbulence, disposing oneself to God's presence, and then surrendering is what we are saying it will take. Kreeft states, "Even the tiny foretaste of heaven that we can all have here on earth by surrendering to God is as much more joyful than the greatest ecstasy sex can give, just as being with your beloved is more joyful than being with her picture."[21]

JOY AS A SECULAR GOAL

From what we have said regarding joy, it is difficult to think of joy as a purely secular reality, that is, something devoid of spirit, transcendence, or otherworldliness. The most non-spiritual thing that perhaps can be said of joy is that it is a function of the human person, that one can experience it apart from any religious faith or belief. Furthermore, joy is something to

[20] Peter Kreeft, "Joy," Op. cit.
[21] Ibid.

16

be espoused and sought after, yet its attainment is elusive. It seems to be the result of a calmed and quieted state whose source wells up from within. And, when it does so, joy can be relished and savored, having far reaching effects on the individual's well-being. These effects have physiological, psychological, and spiritual qualities seen and experienced as lowered heart rate and blood pressure, increased immunity and energy. Psychologically a more positive sense of self, an increased self-esteem, and the healing of relationships can be experienced. Spiritually, there is an increase in self-knowledge and the forces in life that draw oneself to love, compassion, and forgiveness. All, for the moment, seems right with the world.

MINDFULNESS STRICTLY DEFINED

Psychological therapeutic practices acknowledge and use mindfulness as a way of calming and soothing troubled individuals. Mindfulness is defined as,

> "'The quality or state of being mindful,' more specifically, it is 'the practice of maintaining a nonjudgmental state of heightened or complete awareness of one's thoughts, emotions, or experiences on a moment-to-moment basis. It is also such a state of awareness.'"[22]

In short, mindfulness can thus be seen as a conscious mental state that is created by individuals with both their intent to do so and their acting consciously to bring this state about. It lies on the nature — or human side — of the nature/grace continuum we have spoken about previously.[23] Furthermore, the individual is very conscious of the state of awareness that is created. It can begin and end at his own will. In Chapter 4, we will be passing through this membrane between nature (human) and grace (divine) to the grace side of the continuum. It is important to note nevertheless that all the elements of successful mindfulness practice can be helpful as the launch pad for contemplative presence, for without the "nonjudgmental state of heightened or complete awareness of one's thoughts, emotions, or experiences," we are not able to surrender ourselves to a Presence greater and distinct from ourselves.

---

[22] Merriam Webster Dictionary, s.v. "mindfulness," accessed December 5, 2016, http://www.merriam-webster.com.
[23] See page 6 .

JOY, THE FRUIT OF CONTEMPLATIVE PRESENCE

Hopefully, things are becoming a bit clearer regarding joy, from both the side of nature and of grace. From the title of this book, *Moving from Stress to Joy*, we will be making efforts to move from stressful states that result from our day-to-day living to simple stress reducing practices. From there, we will move to practices that dispose us to a greater presence of which we are an integral part. From these efforts, we forge a new way that can be more successful in experiencing both less stress and greater contact with the divine presence. This state of being can become a new "normal." Imagine that! It is most fortunate that we have a connection with God that need not be mediated necessarily by a religion, group, or association. That is, there is an inner part of our being that is beyond ego or personal self. In contemplative prayer, we can choose to identify with that part of ourselves rather than with our bodies or psyches. This growing association, if practiced over time, begins to transform us into that deeper sense of who we are and each step of the deepening results in a greater and deeper joy. It is the reality of our becoming one with the God in whose image we were created and who is constantly drawing us to him. This movement, this deepening joy, is not a creation of our intellect, but it is an experience that is indisputable. It is ours, through no merits of our own, to claim.

GRACE AS ENERGY

When we have quieted our minds and let go of all thinking and distractions, there is an energy within that is contacted. It is very different from the energy we use in thinking, solving a problem, or chatting with another person. In a moment of serene union with nature or mulling over a poem, or hearing the specific movement of a symphony, it is as if you become charged with a spark of energy or emotion. You are actually releasing energy or presence that is always there but is blocked by resistance, stress, distractions, or thinking. Our minds and experiences with the external world block this source of life.

Speaking of this energy, Michael Singer says,

> "The heart is an energy center, and it can open or close...
> This flow of energy comes from the depth of your being. It's
> been called by many names. In ancient Chinese medicine,
> it is called Chi. In yoga, it is called Shakti. In the West, it is
> called Spirit."[24]

---

[24] Michael A. Singer, *The Untethered Soul: The Journey Beyond Yourself*, (Oakland: New Harbinger Publications, Inc., 2007).

The idea of the heart as the energy center calls to mind Catholic devotional practices where the individual prays before an image of the Sacred *Heart* of Jesus or the Immaculate *Heart* of Mary. It appears that in prayer, the union of the one who prays to Jesus or Mary is indeed doing "heart-work." This energy falls on the good and the bad; it is not merited or earned. It is a free gift to all. All it takes to release it is to unbind our own stress and pave the way to dispose us to receive it. Once you taste it and see its extraordinary benefits and the depth of its joy, you have only to continue to choose it — not to allow stress to overtake it — and to remain open and grateful.

GRACE: THE POWER OF CONTEMPLATIVE PRESENCE

In our quieter moments, in moments of unity we may have experienced in a spectacular sunset, the holding of a newborn, or before a work of art — we have experienced such a joy, a taste of heaven. And then we have returned to our stressed-filled environment of family, work, or play and wished for such a moment to return. C.S. Lewis speaks of the power that simply recollecting those moments of unity can bring us back the experience of joy.[25]

But you need not wait for those kinds of moments any longer. You can include such moments in the course of your day through prayer. In a prior work, I have spelled out the three types of prayer and shown the superiority of one.[26] Suffice to name the three as verbal/vocal, meditation, and contemplation. It is through a disposing yourself to the divine presence that you can experience a direct unitive contact with God and the joy of which we have been speaking. Not only is the joy "in the moment," but it also dusts you with a grace that returns you to your activity with a smile on your face and a revived hope in your heart.

Chapter 4 of the present work will deal more extensively with contemplation. We have touched on it here only to make the point that there is a divine reality beneath and within the world of matter. Secondly, there is in the human soul a natural capacity, similarity, and longing for this divine reality.[27]

---

[25] *"That walk I now remembered. It seemed to me that I had tasted heaven then. If only such a moment could return! But what I never realized was that it had returned; that the remembering of that walk had also been desire, and only possession in so far as that kind of desire is itself desirable, is the fullest possession we can know on earth; or rather, because the very nature of Joy makes nonsense of our common distinction between having and wanting. There, to have is to want and to want is to have. Thus the very moment when I longed to be so stabbed again, was itself again such a stabbing."* C.S. Lewis, *Surprised by Joy*, (Orlando: Harcourt Brace Jovanovich, 1955), 166.

[26] Nicholas Amato, *Living in God: Contemplative Prayer and Contemplative Action*, (Bloomington: WestBow Press, 2016), 7ff.

[27] Richard Rohr, "Perennial Wisdom," Richard Rohr's Daily Meditation, January 15, 2017, accessed January 15, 2017, https://cac.org/experience-weekly-summary-2017-01-28/.

If we are able to name our stress, learn ways to quiet it, and dispose ourselves to God's presence, we can effectively unite the psychological and spiritual — nature and grace — to maximize the potential for a truly transformed way of living. This reality is part and parcel of what is called the Perennial Tradition.[28]

The joy of a creator God, a redeemer God, and a God who is closer to our true selves than we could ever imagine, is awaiting our participation. This presence is alluded to in the Hebrew Scriptures and becomes more explicit in the teachings of Jesus reaching their summit in the writings of Paul. Having spoken of the joy that is within us and needs simply to be awakened — thus the title of this book — let us move on to a discussion of the stress that masks that presence, a presence that beckons our awakening.

Reflection Questions for Chapter 2: Christian Joy

- *Describe your own experience of joy.*

- *Where might the joy come from within you, apart from the object that occasions it?*

- *Can you elicit joy when and if you want to? How do you do it?*

---

[28] Ibid.

Chapter 3:
A Preliminary Look at Stress

Stress

The Growth of Stress

The Brain and Stress

Reducing Stress

Stress and the Spiritual Life

WHAT IS STRESS?

Let us begin with a common understanding of what stress is. It is the way that our body responds to what it perceives as a demand or a threat. When we perceive a threat, our bodies mobilize to flee or to fight. It is a very protective response. To do this, our nervous system releases a surge of stress hormones, specifically adrenaline and cortisol. These are the necessary fuels to marshal our body into emergency action. Our heart begins to pound, muscles tighten, blood pressure rises, breath quickens to rush oxygen to the blood stream, and all senses sharpen. All this additional support builds strength and endurance, speeds up our reaction time to the stress, and sharpens our focus. Run or stay and fight, whatever we choose in the end, we are prepared to survive. All this is fine in time of a real danger. However, when it is only a perceived danger or a faraway danger (such as in the news) that we can do nothing about, all this marshaling can have a harmful or dangerous impact on our body and its organs. If the stress is acute and prolonged, the body begins to break down. What started out as a blessing becomes a curse.

We will see that when stress is within our comfort zone, it is actually a help that keeps us focused and energized. It works wonders in getting a job done, completing a project, studying for an exam, or just winning a football game. No question that beyond our comfort zone, stress is no longer helpful and becomes the major reason most folks show up in their doctor's office.

SYMPTOMS OF STRESS

Continuous unmanaged stress will ultimately have an impact on one's health. At the beginning, the symptoms may simply appear as discomfort or a minor nuisance, but they have a way of building on and reinforcing each other, flowering into a major illness or a psychological breakdown of sorts. In her book, *From Stress to Joy,* by Gillian Bethel, the author lists many of both the physical and psychological symptoms of stress.[29]

PHYSICAL

> - Frequent nervous *tics* or muscle spasms
> - Frequent infections and viruses
> - Dry mouth
> - Stiffness, tension, and pain of neck, back, and joints
> - Frequent abdominal pain

---

[29] Gillian Bethel, *From Stress to Joy,* (Roseville: Amazing Facts, Inc., 2004), 317.

- ➤ Frequent indigestion, diarrhea, or constipation
- ➤ Itchy skin
- ➤ Arms crossed or fists clenched while conversing
- ➤ Clutching the steering wheel in traffic
- ➤ Easily startled
- ➤ Frequent headaches
- ➤ Frequent insomnia, fatigue, loss of appetite

PSYCHOLOGICAL

- ➤ Frequent feelings of panic and/or not being in control
- ➤ Frequent depression for no apparent reason
- ➤ Difficulty concentrating on the simplest tasks
- ➤ Frequent impatience
- ➤ Frequent forgetfulness
- ➤ Sudden emotional outbursts and crying spells
- ➤ Frequent worrying or feeling trapped by circumstances
- ➤ Frequent mood swings
- ➤ Frequent irritation over small difficulties
- ➤ Routine tasks become nearly unbearable to accomplish
- ➤ Frequent boredom and/or need for excitement/escapism
- ➤ Increased use of coping mechanisms: alcohol, caffeinated drinks, smoking, drug taking, eating, sleeping, etc.

EARLIEST STAGES OF STRESS CREATION

No one chooses to be stressed. Stress seems to arise from our interaction with the circumstances of our lives. Among them may be an unrealistic deadline to accomplish a task set by my manager, an unreasonable expectation from my spouse, the hotheaded response from one of my children, a traffic jam that will make me late for an important event, and the list goes on. In such situations, we are often sent into a fantasy of how life could be "If only..." and yet we know such "quick fixes" are indeed fantasy or the fix may only be temporary, as we return to our real world of work, play, and living. I would hold that the stress needs to be managed, that is, handled and addressed directly, *and* we need to access a joy that lies deep within the layers of who we really are. Once recaptured, we are able to live with a new sense of understanding and purpose.

There are scores of websites and resources to go to for remedies, but I have found that they often deal with only one aspect of the challenge. It is either managing stress or laying hold of a spiritual presence. Even in the case of the spiritual realm, the suggestions include verbal prayers or scripture passages, both of which are limited in terms of connection. They can keep us in our heads without accessing the core of who we are. What I have found is that having managing techniques is not quite enough to get me over the hump, nor is practicing ineffective prayer very useful. Of course, even with the best accessible contemplative practices, working at disposing myself to God's presence while stressed is very difficult to do. In this regard, it is a question of nature-and-grace, grace-and-nature, and how the two are both important and how they build on one another.[30]

Each of us has a unique way of interacting with situations external to ourselves. We come with different experiences and different emotional resources, so what is stressful for one person may not be stressful for another. A traffic jam may be stressful, but if I have a leisurely afternoon and nothing to do, that same traffic jam will be no big deal. What I hope to offer is the response of others who are on their way to a meeting and will be late because of the traffic delay, but they are able to access specific tools to calm the stress and get through it successfully. Once de-escalated, such individuals may be calm enough even to access a prayer presence that brings waves of joy and delight. This outcome of inner joy is actually what God as creator, redeemer, and sustainer has in mind for us all. It is the joy for which we were created. It is the goal for our life. Living out of this joy is what God wants for us.

A recent poll by the American Psychological Association found 48% of Americans claiming that they were more stressed today than they were only five years ago. Seventy-five percent worry about money and work, which is up from 59% two years before. The correlation between money and stress, because it is so prevalent, may be a good example to illustrate how such a stress grows within us over the years. Do you not find that how you are with money today is how you were with money as a child? I was taught the value of money coming from an immigrant under-classed family and the stress of not having quite enough for "extras," by earning an allowance for house

---

[30] *The Catechism of the Catholic Church*, 1996–1999, 2001–2003.

chores, working my first job stacking bottles behind a diner, and delivering newspapers. That same value for money and the stress of never having quite enough can be seen in my purchase of an automobile, the level of a hotel in which I choose to stay, and how much I am willing to spend for dinner at a restaurant. So, splitting a large dinner bill where I had a low cost entrée and no spirits becomes a moment of some stress. Without managing such stress in these situations, it will eventually exact great costs of anger, resentment, hostility, and eventually avoidance. It should be acknowledged that attitudes toward money could also be derived from one's peers. Here the stress may not be having enough, but not having enough to "keep up with the Joneses."

In the same study, it was found that 45% of adults experienced a decline in health resulting from stress; 95% of all visits to doctors' offices were stress related, and stress has been linked to all six leading causes of death: heart disease, cancer, lung ailments, accidents, liver disease, and suicide.[31] Reported stress levels by generations showed an increase with each generation: 3.5 out of 10 for Matures, 4.3 for Boomers, 5.8 for Xers, and 6.0 for Millennials.[32] While we naturally try to reduce stresses, it is obvious that their persistence over time, coupled with ineffective ways of ridding ourselves of them, begin to take their toll. If we are survivors or if we simply have to put up with the manager whom we see as creating our stress, true, we can quit our job. Most are not able to do that. Thus, over time the level of stress that is felt will come to feel like the normal way we should feel, while the negative effect of the accumulated stresses on our heart, organs, and overall well-being is taking its toll. In Chapter 5, we will consider actual ways to deal with different levels of stress.

HOW STRESS GROWS OVER THE YEARS

Let us fast forward to the present. Life continues to be stressful, and yes, money and spending decisions can cause stress that involve more than just myself. Imagine that! The distinction is, however, that the experience is somewhat different. I have stress-managing tools that I use regularly. There is also a foundational level I can return to — call it a base of reassurance. I am no longer fixed in disillusionment or on a frail foundation of low self-esteem. I've been to the bottom, and now I have tools — a regular practice of contemplative prayer, and several different communities of believers to which I belong. Monthly, I belong to a prayer group, a listening circle, and a priests' support group. Weekly, I have a church community with which to

---

[31] Gillian Bethel. Op. cit., 37.
[32] Ibid.

worship and daily, a friend with whom I share faith and life. Later on in this work, we will see in greater detail how not only to stay the course of joy, but also how to grow and flourish both in stress reduction and in a deeper realization of the grace of presence.

SELF-ESTEEM & STRESS: A CASE IN POINT

In elementary and high school, I had a bit of an inferiority complex. Never measuring up in class, in gym, in looks, in friends, I often felt as if I didn't really belong anywhere. The groups I did manage to edge my way into were not high profile popular groups and included an elementary school friend who was as unpopular as I was, a service club that was not in the esteem category of say the football team, and a fraternity that was at the bottom of the "looked up to" list. So while I did survive, I did so sparingly. When I look at the groups I began to gravitate toward in college, I realize that they were all faith-related in some way. For example, I joined the Newman Club (the Catholic presence on secular college campuses), restoring an old house to become our Newman Center. I began going to Mass on Sunday with students from school. I befriended the chaplain of the Newman Club, and out of all these encounters, a prayer life began to be formed. Eventually, these experiences had me break my engagement to a girl I had known for years, a girl who had also drawn me into regular Catholic worship. Eventually I entered the seminary, and from the day I first set foot on that campus, I was in heaven! The prayer, worship, and community I had experienced in college had lessened the stress, moved me to a deeper experience of God in my life, and filled me with joy. This is not to say the joy made all the stresses disappear. No, the stresses continued, but I was now in touch with a deeper sense of who I was. Prayer, worship, and community were strong antidotes for the clouds that would continue at times to gather. The end of the story, which became the foundation of this book, was acquiring tools for managing stress to calm me and to open myself to God's presence. These tools were to be acquired in my graduate work in psychology and years of applying them to my own life.

RESOURCES ON
STRESS REDUCTION

This is an opportune time to share several important resources on stress reduction.[33] The literature regarding stress is drawn predominantly from psychology and the authors, associations, and online courses available are many. Laurel Mellin is one author I have found most helpful in setting a psychological foundation. Furthermore, her work serves well as a foundation that opens onto the spiritual reality that is part and parcel for healing stressful situations in a permanent and lasting way. This connection struck me several years ago, and I began to offer a series of retreats on the interconnection of the psychological and spiritual aspects stemming from Mellin's foundational work. Again, I see it as nature-and-grace and grace-and-nature. The retreats were attended by contemplative monks, Christian and non-Christian laity, and ministers of other faiths. They were held in monasteries, retreat houses, and parish settings. They were anywhere from a full day to seven day retreats. Thus, they became opportunities to teach the nature-grace connection and to experience its fruits. The results were rather astounding. Using practical techniques to manage stress, moving into contemplative prayer, and then living out of the presence was the key formula.[34]

---

[33] For a more complete list, see the Bibliography, 189.

[34] Nicholas Amato, *Living in God: Contemplative Prayer and Contemplative Action,* (Bloomington: WestBow Press, 2016).

STRESS: GOOD OR BAD?

STRESS CURVE

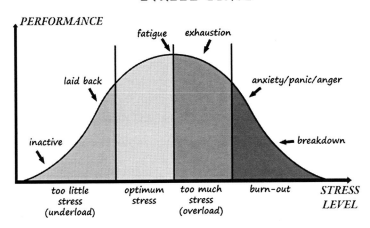

Figure 1 The Stress Curve

Figure 1 presents different levels of stress and how each level impacts performance. The too little stress area speaks of a laid back or inactive posture creating what is called an "underload." At the other extreme are feelings of anxiety, panic, and anger leading to breakdown and eventually burnout. There is, of course, the optimum stress and too much stress areas where most of us live and move, and we modulate back and forth based on our mood, the issues of the day, or the concerns we may have. These two levels would parallel Mellin's Stage 2 of some stress, which uses a tool that checks out one's feelings regarding the stress and her Stage 3 of definite stress, which uses a tool that helps sort out one's emotional response to the stress. While it is worthy of note that some stress maximizes performance, there are limits. Too much stress is not only painful, diminishes work performance, and threatens the quality of our relationships, it can also have an effect on our very DNA.

In a recent study named "The Mindful Workday,"[35] researchers studied the effects of *mindfulness* on workers' increase of focus, improved relationship to their emotions, and the enhancement of their capacity to show compassion. And what was most compelling was to ascertain what was happening within their cells, namely, at the level of gene expression, when comparing pre-test and post-test results over 12 weeks. For 12 weeks, workers were exposed to an hour a week of instruction on mindfulness and compassion.

[35] Parneet Pal, "Stress and Your DNA," February 29, 2016, Mindful, accessed September 19, 2017, https://www.mindful.org/stress-and-your-dna/.

Epigenetics — the branch of science that explores the genes we inherit from our parents that do not change — studies what can change in how those genes get expressed. Such changes can be influenced by lifestyle and environmental elements.[36] Chief among the influences is how we manage or fail to manage our stress. The researchers note that,

> "Though we may inherit a genetic predisposition to various
> chronic diseases — like heart disease, cancer, diabetes,
> anxiety, depression, auto-immune disorders, among others —
> we are empowered through the choices we make each day,
> to keep those from turning into reality."[37]

Chronic disease has been found to be the leading cause of illness and death worldwide. In the U.S., *three out of four of us*[38] will have at least one chronic disease. Just as alarming is the fact that these diseases account for more than 86% of our entire healthcare costs. But there is good news. Eighty to 90% of all chronic disease is *completely preventable* when we pay attention to our lifestyle.[39]

There is a gene set within our DNA that is expressed in an interesting way. It goes up when inflammation is present — as in a "fight or flight" situation of stress — and goes down when immunity is present. Thus, a decreased expression in the gene set will create the conditions for a healthier result. The expression of this gene set was compared before and after the 12 weeks of the experiment. It was found that the expression actually did change over time.[40]

> ➤ There was a significantly lower expression of inflammatory genes, and greater expression of genes boosting immunity.

> ➤ There were statistically significant improvements in their psychological and social wellbeing

> ➤ There was a trend for a greater reported sense of connection over the 12 weeks

> ➤ There was an upward trend in levels of mindful awareness (the ability to pay attention to the present without getting lost in past or future).

---

[36] Ibid.

[37] Ibid.

[38] "Chronic Disease Prevention and Health Promotion," Centers for Disease Control and Prevention, last updated September 13, 2017, accessed September 19, 2017, https://www.cdc.gov/chronicdisease/.

[39] "Healthy Living is the best revenge: Findings from the European Prospective Investigation Into Cancer and Nutrition – Potsdam study," US National Library of Medicine National Institutes of Health, accessed September 19, 2017, https://www.ncbi.nlm.nih.gov/pubmed/19667296.

[40] https://www.mindful.org/stress-and-your-dna/, Op. cit.

It is heartening to know the effect mindfulness meditation can have on what might first appear to be a negative inherited influence on our wellbeing. Our dispositions at birth may not have to be our destiny against psychological and spiritual flourishing.

Elizabeth Scott comes a bit closer to where we are heading in the Nature/Grace or Stress/Joy equation. In an article entitled "Use Spirituality for Stress Relief,"[41] she begins by affirming that those who incorporate spirituality tend to fare better with stress. Her techniques work whether you are part of a spiritual community, church, prayer group, or not. Her advice is to pray often, express gratitude, be intrinsically oriented, maintain optimism, and find the lesson that is to be learned. There is no question that the more we are connected to the divine, the safer and more reassured we will feel. This will be an important consideration in Chapter 4 on contemplation as a very specific kind of prayer and deeper than meditation. Prayer, in any of its forms, has shown to lower blood pressure and heart rate and heighten immunity. The calm that comes over a person is undeniable. On a personal note, I find that when I go to my internist for my annual checkup, I always arrive early and sit in prayer for 15 minutes. It is amazing how different a reading the assistant gets from when I come in from a morning's rush hour of traffic. Would you believe 20–25 points difference! Such calming not only puts the present stress to rest, but it also prepares you for the next perception of stress as well.

Expressing gratitude to God is a tried and true way of reducing stress, for it puts you in a different frame of mind that moves from stressor-focused to a focus on other things in the mind or an environment that boosts a positive outlook. It could be the smallest of things like the weather, something that you are looking forward to during the day, a plan you have in the future, or something as simple as the ability to breathe. Make this a regular habit at the end of your day, and two marvelous things begin to happen. You will begin to see more and more things for which you are grateful, things that largely went unnoticed, and second, you will begin to experience gratitude in the moment — as the gratitude is taking place, rather than simply in your recollecting it at the end of the day. I have often encouraged folks I have for spiritual guidance to recall five things for which they are grateful before laying their head on the pillow and to jot them into a little spiral bound notebook on their bed stand or, if they already keep a journal, to enter them there. The only rule is that they cannot ever repeat a blessing. This forces them to look for new ones and, as they do so, the blessings shift to smaller and smaller ones that would have been overlooked in the past. The list can serve as a concrete pick-me-up by reviewing it for the past week when things are becoming stressful and anxiety is beginning to build. This will also be helpful as a pathway for disposing yourself to contemplative prayer.

[41] Elizabeth Scott, "Use Spirituality for Stress Relief," Very Well, last updated July 13, 2016, accessed December 9, 2016, https://www.verywell.com/use-spirituality-for-stress-relief-3144819.

Being intrinsically oriented is another way Scott suggests reducing the stress you are feeling. Remaining fixed on God, maintaining the faith that has gotten you through tougher times in the past, and surrendering to the divine will are all part of this intrinsic orientation. Extrinsic resources would include touching base with friends of the same faith, a prayer group, or a worshipping community. Research indicates that we experience greater benefits from being intrinsically oriented.

Maintaining a sense of optimism is also an important consideration for stress reduction. Just this morning, I had some car trouble with my brand new automobile. I was scheduled to leave town to be with a friend who is critically ill. It began to rain. I had to take the car in to the dealership for emergency service. Wow! How tense, how stressed did I feel? Lots! I began thinking of a modified schedule: on the drive to the dealership I could complete the audio book I am enjoying, and, during the time at the dealership, I would work on this manuscript. Am I an optimist? You bet, I am! It is easy to see how optimists tend to experience less stress than pessimists or, for that matter, realists. There is an unspoken assumption on our part that we can get through this trial; we can expect good things to happen. As a result, stress-producing events are seen as insignificant setbacks that can be overcome. Positive events are proof of further good things to take place, and the risk is worth the wait. In addition, research bears out that optimists are more proactive with the management of stress, and they favor approaches that reduce or eliminate stressors and their emotional consequences. Optimists work harder at stress management, so they're less stressed.[42]

Scott's final strategy is to find the lesson within a stressful situation. Here, along with many mystics, she recommends that those who are spiritual have the added benefit of looking at stressful situations as tests of endurance in the name of faith or to view them as God's proving ground. Scripture itself attests to this:

> ➤ Psalm 26:2 — "Test me, Lord, and try me, examine my heart and my mind."

> ➤ Psalm 66:10 — "For you, God, tested us; you refined us like silver."

> ➤ Psalm 139:23 — "Search me, God, and know my heart; test me and know my anxious thoughts."

> ➤ Proverbs 17:3 — "The crucible for silver and the furnace for gold, but the Lord tests the heart."

---

[42] Elizabeth Scott, "The Benefits of Optimism," Very Well, last modified April 28, 2016, accessed December 10, 2016, https://www.verywell.com/the-benefits-of-optimism-3144811.

This distinction is good for seeing stress regarding a particular situation as a test, making the stressful situation less threatening, ominous, or unwanted. Thus, there would be less of a reaction, which could open the way for a more effective, less emotional response. After all, it *is* the way God operates with those whom he loves. The alternative is thus opened to overall greater growth.

We have now clearly moved from stress to ways of coping with stress, both psychological, to some bordering on the spiritual. This movement forward, in the present book, is intentional, for we support and are looking to uncover the essential role that God, prayer, and specifically contemplative prayer, play in the movement from stress to joy. Along this continuum, we become accustomed to feeling "at home" at any given point. It simply becomes what we're used to, what seems to have become the norm. It can be referred to as a "set-point."

CREATION OF THE SET-POINT

Set-point is a term that is familiar to weight reduction. It states that,

> "The set-point is a level of body fat…that your body will tend to return to, regardless of any changes you make to your diet or activity level. The set-point is a function of physiological mechanisms — such as how well you build muscle or store and burn fat, among others — but also central mechanisms in the brain which regulate bodily processes and behaviors. It's those central systems that are of interest, since they regulate the behavior of muscle, fat, and, unsurprisingly, you (you in the sense of personal identity)."[43]

It is as if our body has an internal thermostat. When you diet below your set point, it will become evident, for you will consistently be hungry. However, at levels of leanness that lie outside the internally programmed parameters, your hunger will change. We are told that we can out-willpower the drive, but it is not going to be easy.[44] Regrettably, the body will always win, and the dieters eat themselves back to the level of fat with which the body is "happy."

While this balancing out, also called homeostasis, may look like a liability, it is actually the way the body strives for some stability. Homeostasis is necessary to remain alive. "Most everything in the body has a set-point of

---

[43] "The Cortical Lottery: Dopamine and the Activity Set-Point," Myosynthesis, last modified March 3, 2011, accessed December 10, 2016, www.myosynthesis.com/cortical-lottery-dopamine-activity-setpoint.

[44] Ibid.

some kind," remarks the Myosynthesis website.[45] It is also known that humans have genetically-governed happiness set points. Events can make us very happy, such as receiving a pay raise. They can also be the cause of sadness, such as being laid off at work. Whatever they may be, they are often seen as temporary, and we bounce back to our original set point, what is sometimes called our *affective style*.[46] I will hold that it is different, however, when the grace side of our equation is supplied in the form of contemplative prayer. From the "nature" side of the equation, we are on a bit of a seesaw. Sometimes we are up; sometimes we are down — gains and losses, gains and losses — but always anchored to the central crossbeam of the seesaw, remaining more or less in one place. Your baseline happiness and affective style are a function of the genes you received from your parents. It can be shown that change begins in our thoughts. The behaviors flow from those thoughts and impacts change in the brain.[47] As a final outcome, it changes how we can respond to stress. The brain does influence thought, but thought also influences the brain and to a greater degree than we have once believed.

By nature, I see myself as a survivor, a perfectionist, and I have been known to have some compulsive traits. When hosting overnight guests, for example, I find that preparing their lodging, planning menus, and creating social things to do can be somewhat stressful. In Figure 1, that would be activities in the area of optimum stress and moving toward experiencing fatigue. Simple sketching out of a plan with remote, proximate, and immediate goals keeps me from hitting fatigue or, even worse, moving into the area of too much stress and exhaustion. One way I keep from moving to fatigue would be to include time for a nap in the very plan. In the end, reorganizing priorities, asking someone at home to lend a helping hand, or simplifying the menu are all strategies to keep me out of the "anxiety/panic/anger" area. Being a survivor keeps my shoulder to the plough. "Where do prayer and presence enter into the stress reduction equation?" you ask. No day begins or ends without silent reflection on who I am and what I will be doing, and who am I and what did I do that day. It grounds and works in conjunction with all of the stress-reducing efforts aforementioned. We will see this in greater detail after we have considered contemplation.

---

[45] Ibid.

[46] Ibid.

[47] Bruce McEwen is a neuro-endocrinologist and stress researcher at Rockefeller University. He has studied the central factors of stress response and demonstrated how it is, quite literally, all in the mind. Your body affects your thought and changes your behavior. In turn, these changes emerge as a stress response in your body.

CHANGING THE SET-POINT

Even in light of the seeming intransigence of a set-point, it is possible to change it. It must be more than willpower, however, willpower is an important component for success. No one can change your set-point of stress for you, although having someone with whom to share your goal and be accountable goes a long way.

This changing of set-point came home to me recently regarding a close priest friend of mine. As the pastor of a very large parish of 4,300 families and 11,000 people, and eight Sunday Masses, he continued to chug along as a very effective and well-loved pastor. He did this for ten years at this one parish and throughout those years, I noticed he was continuously having to meet deadlines, be available 24/7, and struggling to take time for himself for exercise. Last June 30th, he retired from this pastoral position and has settled down into helping out in two parishes on weekends, having only a total of two Masses any weekend, leading an occasional retreat or day of recollection, and seeing four individuals for Spiritual Direction each week. He reports that he is now sleeping better, feels little or no stress, and is experiencing greater overall well-being. As his friend, I can see he looks and acts more relaxed, and he is more open to a broader array of alternatives regarding what to do together, where to go, what to watch, or where to eat.

While we are not all able to retire, nor do we want to, there are other ways to change your set-point as to what levels of stress feels normal. Knowing and managing the level at which you are and accessing the power of silence can lead to meaningful change, for as you increasingly experience inner joy, it becomes a place you want to go more often and spend more time. Eventually, the stress and the joy stand out in sharp contrast to one another, and a craving for the joy begins to take hold. You are now moving from an occasional shot of joy to savoring gentle sips of joy that last longer and longer. This is not to say that you will live full-time in that state, but it is to say you will know the taste and the way to get there. It is where God wants us very much to be. It is the fullness of joy that Jesus prayed for before the Last Supper.

In his bestselling book, *The Power of Habit: Why We Do What We Do in Life and Business,* Charles Duhigg, an investigative reporter for *The New York Times* speaks of how our habits form and how they can change. He states,

> "This process within our brains is a three-step loop. First, there is a cue, a trigger that tells your brain to go into automatic mode and which habit to use. Then there is the routine, which can be physical or mental or emotional. Finally,

there is a reward, which helps your brain figure out if this particular loop is worth remembering for the future: THE HABIT LOOP."[48]

The loop looks something like this:

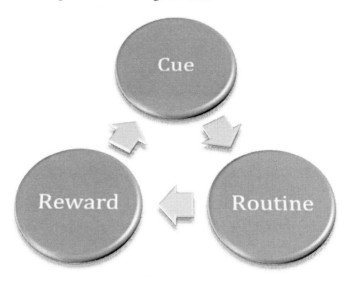

Figure 2 The Habit Loop

In order to change a habit, or for our understanding, to reset your set-point, you must keep the old cue and deliver the old reward, but insert a new routine. Perhaps a personal example would help. Ten years ago, if I did not have an evening meeting at my parish, I would always have a cocktail before dinner. This preference eventually developed into a habit. When I retired from being a pastor and having evening meetings, the daily cocktail became ingrained. It was a habit complete with a cue — setting sun, day is done — and routine — chilling the cocktail glass, getting out the olive and spirits, selecting the nuts or snacks, and the reward — relaxation and a bit of euphoria. In repeating this over several months, I developed the set-point of the euphoria that the practice carried with it. Having a cocktail every evening became the new "normal." What I realized had me stuck was the good feeling it gave me, the reward. This is not meant to say that a cocktail is not a good thing, nor do I want to sound puritanical.

Because I was already praying in silence every morning and evening, I began to compare the positive feelings such prayer brought me with the feelings delivered by the evening cocktail. They were similar, yet different.

---

[48] Charles Duhigg, *The Power of Habit: Why We Do What We Do in Life and Business,* (New York: Random House Trade Paperbacks, 2012), 19.

Clearly the silence and prayer won out over the cocktail by comparison. The old cue of wanting to relax a bit before dinner remained, but I now had a new routine, namely, preparing for contemplative prayer rather than mixing a cocktail, and the old reward of euphoria, though the same, was a deeper, fuller "high."

Willpower is like a muscle in your arm; you have to work at it, and it does get tired so that after a while it is ready to quit. Duhigg holds that the thing that moves a new behavior from merely an exercise of pure willpower to a full-fledged habit is the eventual craving in one's mind for the reward achieved by the new routine. In my own case, the craving for the deeper satisfaction I received from contemplative prayer now finds me, after 10 years, no longer drinking spirits, save wine at Eucharist. Figure 3 adds the key factor of craving. If sheer acts of willpower are to become an acquired habit, where less effort and greater motivation to act positively are experienced, it will take developing a sense of craving. When you crave something, it is much easier to choose it. Doing so time and time again creates the habit.

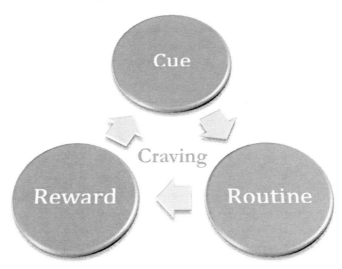

Figure 3 The Craving Brain

Willpower was needed initially, but the craving got me out of the "willing" into craving the deeper value of God's abiding presence.

COMMON STRESSES

In studies done by the American Psychological Association with over 1,000 people in 2007, 2008, 2009, and 2010, participants were asked to select from a list of things people say cause stress in their lives. They were also asked to indicate how significant a source of stress the item was for them. The top stressors were money, work, the economy, family responsibilities, relationships, personal health concerns, housing costs, job stability, health problems affecting the family, and personal safety, in that order.[49] (See Figure 4 on page 39)

COMMON WAYS
OF REDUCING STRESSES

In that same study for the years 2008, 2009, and 2010, participants were asked which of the following items helped them manage their stress: listen to music, exercise or walk, spend time with friends or family, read, watch TV more than two hours a day, and pray. Sadly, from our perspective, praying was just above playing video games or surfing the Internet.[50] My question would be what was meant by "praying" and how effectively were subjects disposing themselves to God's presence. Also it is worth noting that many of the ways of reducing stress mentioned, particularly listening to music, walking, and reading, could be ways of moving one into the silence. These will be further considered in our next chapter. (See Figure 5 on page 40)

---

[49] "Stress in America," America Psychological Association, accessed December 12, 2017, https://www.apa.org/news/press/releases/stress/2010/national-report.pdf, 8.
[50] "Stress in America," Op. cit., 11.

Causes of Stress
% Somewhat/Very Significant

■ 2007 ■ 2008 ■ 2009 ■ 2010

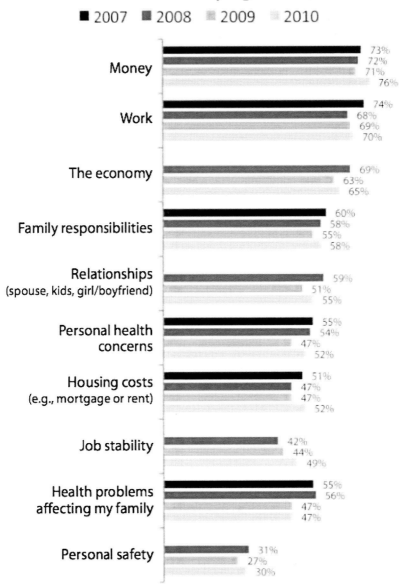

Money	73% / 72% / 71% / 76%
Work	74% / 68% / 69% / 70%
The economy	69% / 63% / 65%
Family responsibilities	60% / 58% / 55% / 58%
Relationships (spouse, kids, girl/boyfriend)	59% / 51% / 55%
Personal health concerns	55% / 54% / 47% / 52%
Housing costs (e.g., mortgage or rent)	51% / 47% / 47% / 52%
Job stability	42% / 44% / 49%
Health problems affecting my family	55% / 56% / 47% / 47%
Personal safety	31% / 27% / 30%

BASE: All respondents 2007 (n=1848); 2008 (n=1791); 2009 (n=1568); 2010 (n=1134)
Q625 Below is a list of things people say cause stress in their lives. For each one, please indicate how significant a source of stress it is in your life.

Figure 4 Causes of Stress

Stress Management

■ 2008 ■ 2009 ■ 2010

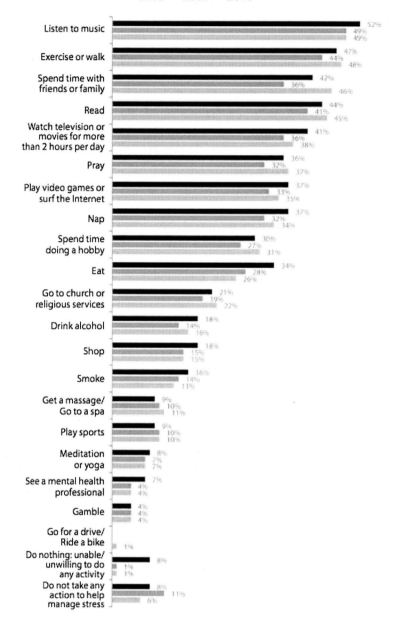

	2008	2009	2010
Listen to music	52%	49%	49%
Exercise or walk	47%	44%	48%
Spend time with friends or family	42%	36%	46%
Read	44%	41%	45%
Watch television or movies for more than 2 hours per day	41%	36%	38%
Pray	36%	32%	37%
Play video games or surf the Internet	37%	33%	35%
Nap	37%	32%	34%
Spend time doing a hobby	30%	27%	31%
Eat	34%	28%	26%
Go to church or religious services	21%	19%	22%
Drink alcohol	18%	14%	16%
Shop	18%	15%	15%
Smoke	16%	14%	13%
Get a massage/ Go to a spa	9%	10%	11%
Play sports	9%	10%	10%
Meditation or yoga	8%	7%	7%
See a mental health professional	7%	4%	4%
Gamble	4%	4%	4%
Go for a drive/ Ride a bike		1%	
Do nothing: unable/ unwilling to do any activity	8%	1%	1%
Do not take any action to help manage stress	8%	11%	6%

BASE: All respondents 2008 (n=1791); 2009 (n=1568); 2010 (n=1134)
Q965 Do you do any of the following to help manage stress? Please select all that apply.

Figure 5 Stress Management

FIVE SIMPLE STEPS
TO STRESS REDUCTION

The website BeBrainFit.com[51] offers five simple tips to stop stress and its negative impact on your brain. I cite them to show how they reinforce the connection between nature and grace, of which we have been speaking.

- ➤ Eat a diet high in antioxidant-rich foods like fruit, vegetables, dark chocolate, and green tea.

- ➤ Get daily physical exercise.

- ➤ Begin a daily meditation practice. Meditation not only reduces stress, it's a proven way to keep your brain young. Meditation is also the best tool for learning how to master your thoughts. Stress does not come from events in your life as much as it comes from your thoughts — your automatic negative reactions and cognitive distortions — about these events.

- ➤ Try mind-body relaxation techniques.

- ➤ Look into taking an herbal remedy.

While chronic stress may be a part of your life, there are ways offered by the medical community for reducing its negative impact on the functioning of your brain.

We are not going to discuss here the advantages that diet, physical exercise, or herbal remedies have on stress reduction. These advantages are part of a Priest Wellness Program I created several years ago and remain as important factors in contributing to overall wellness.[52] Nevertheless, a word needs to be said about the other two factors for stress reduction, namely, meditation and mind-body relaxation techniques. They play an important part in the process, not only of stress reduction, but also in preparing for the experience of grace, the second half of the equation. For unless we tap into a deep resource that is the very ground of our being and unless we can access what is very much part of our spiritual DNA, the stress reduction will not endure. For me, it is all about stress reduction (nature) and reclaiming the joy (grace) that makes it a life enhancing change.

There is no question that meditation has a unique way of calming our minds and putting us at rest. And as the authors of BrainFit say, it does help keep your brain young. I continue to agree with them that it is an excellent way

---

[51] Deanne Alban, "12 Effects of Chronic Stress on Your Brain," Be Brain Fit, accessed December 7, 2016, https://bebrainfit.com/effects-chronic-stress-brain/.

[52] The Mepkin Priest Wellness Program is a week of intensive training in prayer, nutrition, exercise, and community for Catholic priests and began at Mepkin Trappist Abbey in South Carolina.

to learn how to master your thoughts. Whether you are a compulsive worrier, an anxious participant, or a constant planner, thoughts and their control have to be mastered. When we deal with contemplative prayer, several ways to gain control of thoughts will be proffered, but our excitement will not end with simply a calmed mind. This control will be the prelude to disposing us to a presence that will make a long-term difference when we consider handling stress prayerfully in Chapter 7. A second issue that is raised in the preceding five stress reduction tips is the encouragement to use mind-body relaxation techniques. This is an excellent suggestion. In Chapter 4, we will see how acquiring the art of deep breathing and using a simple biofeedback technique will be part of an escalator to take us to the depths of inner silence. This conviction of how natural psychological techniques can help dispose us to God's presence were borne out in my years as a Spiritual Integrator at St. Luke Institute. The combination of psychology and spirituality working together in the life of a believer could bring the individual to regaining the joy he first experienced in making his solemn vows or on the day of his ordination.

MEDITATION OR CONTEMPLATION?

We have mentioned contemplation as a way to pray and are clearly favoring it among the other ways to pray. Perhaps a description of the other two types of prayer and a word of clarification is in order. In the West, we divide prayer into verbal/vocal prayer, meditation, and contemplation.[53] Verbal/vocal prayer would encompass rote prayers, read prayer, devotions, Liturgy of the Hours, the rosary, and the Psalms. Meditation is the use of the imagination to conjure a scene from Sacred Scripture, nature, poetry, music, or work of art. We place ourselves in the scene and create an interaction with persons of a higher power that the scene elicits. Contemplation is achieving a state of awareness, with nothing added on our part. No thoughts, no distractions, no feelings. We simply let go and allow ourselves to enter God's presence. The term *meditation* is a bit equivocal, that is, it means two very different things depending on the person to whom you are speaking. In the East, when they speak of meditation, they mean the reality we speak of, as contemplation. The difference is that for us, meditation involves active engagement of the mind in a scene, incorporating all the five senses and drawing oneself into the scene. Of course, the creation of the scene is both dependent upon and limited by the imaginative acumen of the meditator. Meditation, in the East, is a suspending of the mind's thoughts, images, and concerns. It is allowing oneself to be in the void with nothing added by the individual.

---

[53] Teresa of Ávila, *The Way of Perfection*, translated and edited by E. Allison Peers, (London: Doubleday, 1946), 153ff, 193ff.

However, whether it is contemplation for the Westerner or meditation for the Easterner, one difference still remains, namely, the Christian is in the space of "no-thought" to encounter God as present face-to-face, as scripture attests.[54] The person from the East is there to encounter the void.

BRAIN STATES

It may be helpful to ground meditation and contemplation in the physiology of the brain, that is, what is going on in my brain when I meditate or contemplate? The *Tools for Wellness* website states that there are four brain states known as Beta, Alpha, Theta, and Delta. Each state contributes to various activities of the mind. Thus, the Beta state allows for alertness, concentration, and cognition. The Alpha state makes relaxation, visualization, and creativity possible. Of special interest to us is the Theta state, which makes possible meditation, intuition, and memory. In this state, you are very close to sleep, but not quite there. This state *Tools for Wellness* says is,

> "Where magic happens in the crucible of your own neurological activity. Theta brings forward heightened receptivity, flashes of dreamlike imagery, inspiration, and your long-forgotten memories. Theta can bring you deep states of meditation. A sensation of 'floating.' And, because it is an expansive state, in Theta, you may feel your mind expand beyond the boundaries of your body."[55]

In contrast to the prior three states, Delta brainwaves are slow, loud brainwaves. Generated in deepest meditation and dreamless sleep, they suspend external awareness. Healing and regeneration are stimulated in this state, and this is why deep restorative sleep is so essential to our regeneration and healing.[56] Rather than such "brain states," you can also think of "states of the brain." From this perspective, we would argue that "brain states" are patterns of neural firing, reflecting the electrical face of the brain, whereas "states of the brain" are the modulating of neural activity that represent more the chemical face of the brain.

The goal to make liberating prayer possible would be to move to the Theta state of consciousness where meditation, as an action of the one who prays, can be transformed into a sense of free floating. Here grace can have its most effective impact.

---

[54] "The Lord spoke to you face to face out of the fire on the mountain." Deuteronomy 5:4 and "Look to the Lord and his strength; seek his face always." Psalms 105:4.

[55] "The Four Brain States," Tools for Wellness, accessed December 7, 2016, http://www.toolsforwellness.com/brainstates.html.

[56] "What Are Brainwaves?" Brainworks, accessed September 19, 2017, http://www.brainworksneurotherapy.com/what-are-brainwaves.

PSYCHOLOGICAL JOY VERSUS SPIRITUAL JOY

Moving from stress, let us turn now to consider the state of joy and see how psychological joy might differ from spiritual joy or if they are one and the same. There is an assumption that when one has removed all levels of stress, the individual sinks delightfully into State 1 which is the state of Joy. When in this state, the individual is counseled to feel compassion for you and for others and compassion for all that lives (wisdom/love). If you are not able to feel such compassion, you are not in a state of joy. It appears that this state is a psychological state of well-being: feeling good about yourself, and all seems right with the world. It is these secure emotional attachments to yourself that anchor you with a sense of inner strength, goodness, and wisdom. We will see in our next chapter on contemplation that joy, rather than being what is left when stress is effectively managed for the moment, is more the intimate union of the Lover and the Beloved, God and the one in prayer. It is really focused in mutuality and union. It is clearly a relationship. And not only is it the result of contemplative presence, but the shared love, the mutuality that is a resource that can be accessed in any of the states of stress. This is where spirituality plays such a central role in stress reduction. This is not to say the tools of State 5 (Definitely Stressed) and State 3 (Somewhat Stressed) will not help as well. Used together, the tools *and* the presence become indomitable partners in psychological and spiritual health. I would not be honest if I did not share where I would end up if I did not use the coping skills for Stages 3 and 5. Part of my own coping panoply involves uncontrolled eating of leftovers, going for the box of chocolate or the bags of nuts. I have developed alternatives to choosing destructive or less than growth-full alternatives. A few of the alternatives I find helpful are doing some brisk walking, chewing a piece of gum, or eating an orange, as a compromise. A written dialogue with the temptation, as if it were an individual, has also been very helpful at times. Such a practice feeds into my objectifying the temptation and competing with it and winning! Thus, in addition to the tools, I also have specific activities that I can employ to protect myself from having stress take over my life. A third and final resource is to lay hold of God's healing and sustaining presence in my life.

CHRISTIAN JOY, THE GIFT THAT FLOWS FROM PRESENCE

I have asserted what I believe joy is and what it is not. It is not what is left over when stress is reduced. It is not only the fruit of healthy self-esteem. I like to think of it as the fruit of our experience of being or resting within God. And in contemplative prayer, we are able to leave ego behind and bask in God's presence, so much so, that we are one with that presence. What draws us to it inexorably is the longing for the divine presence. What flows from it is pure joy. To experience it is beyond words. Let us now turn to a consideration of contemplation as a primary way to recapture the promise of joy that is already there awaiting us.

Reflection Questions for Chapter 3: A Preliminary Look at Stress

> ❧ *What are the symptoms of your own stress?*

> ❧ *Do you ever experience stress as helpful? If so, how?*

> ❧ *How do you compare your own stress levels with those of other family members? With those of folks with whom you work?*

Chapter 4: Contemplation

Joy
1. Christian Joy: What it is
2. Christian Joy: How to get there
3. We're Not Pelagians

Examples
4. Magic Moments
5. A Time and a Place for Contemplation

History
6. A Thumbnail History of Contemplation
7. Foundational Documents for Contemplative Prayer
8. Teresa of Ávila's Contribution as the Gold Standard
9. Three Cistercian Founders
10. Contribution of John Main

Going In and Coming Out
11. The Call of the Deep
12. Going In: Attention versus Intention
13. What Goes on in the "Space" of "No-Space"?
14. What Comes Out of This "Space" of "No-Space"?
15. Going In to Contemplation; Coming Out
16. Meditation Is Not Contemplation

Alternatives to Contemplative Prayer
17. If Contemplation Isn't for You
18. Pray as You Can, Not as You Ought

Pitfalls: Dualism and Dialectical Thinking
19. Dialectical Thinking and the Joy of Centering Prayer
20. Ego Consciousness and Contemplation

Liabilities and Blessings
21. True Self-False Self
22. Gifts Received in Contemplation
23. The Fruits of Contemplation
24. Effects of Meditation and Contemplation on Our DNA
25. Effect of "Letting Go" of Thoughts
26. Childhood Caveats

Mystics
27. Secular and Religious Mystics
28. Mystics of Many Colors

Moving Toward the Next Chapter

Transitioning to Chapter

CHRISTIAN JOY: WHAT IT IS

Christian joy is an abiding and empowering presence of Jesus to us. At its best, it is the promise of the Lord to us as individuals and as a community. But it is more than a promise; it is empowerment in the here and now and to have that promise fulfilled. Think of it as the promise of parents to you as a teenager who would give you the old family car when you turned 18. Forget that it's the family jalopy and, instead, consider the "promise of joy" that is awaiting you! Let us recall for a moment what that promise from the Lord is. He expresses it in the Gospel of John just before he is to face his passion.[57]

> "Abide in me, and I in you. As the branch cannot bear fruit by itself, unless it abides in the vine, neither can you, unless you abide in me. I am the vine; you are the branches. He who abides in me, and I in him, he it is that bears much fruit, for apart from me you can do nothing...As the Father has loved me, so have I loved you; abide in my love. If you keep my commandments, you will abide in my love, just as I have kept my Father's commandments and abide in his love. These things I have spoken to you, *that my joy may be in you, and that your joy may be full* [emphasis added]...You did not choose me, but I chose you and appointed you that you should go and bear fruit and that your fruit should abide; so that whatever you ask the Father in my name, he may give it to you. This I command you, to love one another."

That presence will be experienced as joy in its fullness. More importantly, that joy in us will overflow into a love and care for self and others. This idea of overflowing into a love and care for self and others will be covered as an important part of Chapter 6 where stress will have been managed, contemplative presence experienced, and we will see the flowering of both in our relationship with others.

Two religious mystics that have something to say about this joy are Julian of Norwich and Teresa of Ávila. Julian, who experienced moments of God's direct revelation and perfect union with him, said, "Between God and the soul there is no between."[58] Teresa of Ávila attested that in her moments in contemplation, the Almighty became one with her nature and transformed her into himself, which brought about a union of creator and creature, where the Lord delighted in her soul and her soul delighted in the Lord.[59] From my own

---

[57] John 15:4-17, (Revised Standard Version).

[58] Julian of Norwich, "Julian of Norwich Quotes," AZ Quotes, accessed January 15, 2017, http://www.azquotes.com/author/17697-Julian_of_Norwich.

[59] Jordan Aumann, O.P., "St. Teresa's Teaching on the Grades of Prayer," Catholic Culture, accessed January 17, 2017, www.catholicculture.org/culture/library/view.cfm?id=7725.

experience with contemplative prayer, limited though it be, there is a complete loss of the sense of time and a sweetness enjoyed, without noticing or having any considerations about it. It is more a basking, resting in, and savoring.

CHRISTIAN JOY: HOW TO GET THERE

Jesus perhaps put it most succinctly when he told us how to pray most effectively: "But when you pray, go into your room and shut the door and pray to your Father who is in secret; and your Father who sees in secret will reward you."[60]

The "how" then has to do with disposing oneself, seeking silence and seclusion, getting out of the flow of life, paradoxically, to become one with the flow of life. So what seems apparent is completely the opposite. This should not surprise us. Reason and thinking do not exercise much control in matters of the heart, especially when it comes to love, presence, and communion.

In this chapter, we will look closely at the practices and tools that can get us out of control so *God* can be in control. These practices and tools allow us to be active in our disposition over and over again, for there is no point where one arrives and remains in the presence, even though it is God who is encountered. The "holding power" though divine, requires our letting go, surrendering as a steady state. Any returning to control, thinking, or even consciously considering the delight, whisks us away, out of our hearts and back into our heads.

WE'RE NOT PELAGIANS[61]

Yes, we do make an effort at disposing ourselves, but it is not our effort that makes, forces, or controls God to be present to us in any way. God is present in every moment; it is we who do not connect. You might liken it to broadcast waves in the air: always there, never seen, not apparent to the senses. What it takes is a receiver of some sort — a human being in the analogy — and a person that is tuned into the precise frequency, before what is present and unseen can be heard, seen, experienced, and enjoyed. It is all about practices to dispose oneself to the divine presence, and to continue the analogy, to set up the audio or video receiver, as the believer, to be on the correct frequency to see and experience what is really there.

---

[60] Matthew 6:6, (Revised Standard Version).

[61] According to his opponents, Pelagius taught that moral perfection was attainable in this life without the assistance of divine grace through human free will. In condemning the heresy, the Council of Carthage in 418 stated that without God's grace it is not merely more difficult, but absolutely impossible to perform good works.

MAGIC MOMENTS

Not all time spent in contemplation happens during spans of time that are set aside for this type of prayer. James Finley speaks of it more as a way of life where, "To contemplate means to observe carefully to pay attention. Throughout the day, things catch our eye and we momentarily contemplate them."[62] There is an intuitive sense in the believer or the person who has experienced such instances before, that God is the very ground of our being and of all that exists. Whatever shimmered or caught our attention in the moment becomes a kind of portal to encountering the divine, a diving board into the pool of Being. Because of the way the object holds and captures, first our attention, then our longing, and finally our very selves, we become one in the experience and can remain there indefinitely. For the one so captured, it is often someone's calling to us, or a loud disturbance that wakes us from our reverie. What we have experienced is an outpouring of God and the joy of union. Finley continues,

> "In these moments, we intuitively use the word God for the infinity of the primordial preciousness we, in such moments, realize ourselves to be one with. In these moments we realize that nothing is missing anywhere and what fools we are to worry so."[63]

In my seminary days, I remember the maxims "Maintain a state of recollection" and "Eternalize the present moment." Outside of formal times set aside for prayer, they went a long way in getting in touch and staying in touch with deeper levels of experience that seemed to pop up many times in a day. "Maintaining" and "Eternalizing" with awareness, we can experience more often and more deeply the divine presence in every breath we take, every beat of our heart. Unfortunately, the world and all its allurements keep us from doing that by seizing our attention and ultimately selling us something.

Magic moments can also be times remembered. Here, the memory serves to bring back a past occurrence that gives joy or pleasure in the moment. We sink into it and allow it to envelope us. The memory may fade, leaving only the joy that it brought, but re-experienced. One such memory I have is the picture embedded in my memory when I was walking down a dirt road as a boy of 11 in cutoffs with a fishing pole in my hand and a peanut butter and jelly sandwich and a thermos of water in a cloth bag tied to my jeans, anticipating a full day away from my family in the Catskill Mountains of New York State. When the picture fades, the joy of freedom, solitude, and adventure linger. A second such memory fills a bit more of my affiliative needs.

---

[62] Adapted from James Finley, exclusive Center for Action and Contemplation Living School curriculum, Unit 1.

[63] Ibid.

It's playing Monopoly every New Year's Eve as teenagers at our cousins' home until the wee hours of the morning with my siblings and cousins. When the memory dwindles, the savoring of the joy of being part of an extended family, feeling safe, and loved are savored for as long as I would want to remain there.

A TIME AND A PLACE FOR CONTEMPLATION

We need not wait for or create magic moments to experience contemplation. We can choose a place and set a time in the day to pray in this way. For many it is morning and evening, sitting in silence for a length of time without having the need to recall old memories or rely on magic moments. It is no accident that such times devoted to contemplative prayer have more to do with the heart than the head; with gazing rather than looking; with being, rather than doing; with awareness, than thinking. The heart has the capacity to move us beyond being right about ideology, controlling another person, or forcing our will on others. All forms of verbal/vocal prayer, meditation, and contemplation can get us along that 18-inch journey from our head to our heart, but contemplation can do it most effectively. In the end, a surrendered heart is able to balance out beautifully our ever present, calculating mind. It is no easy task, however. It requires a continuing effort to dispose us to the movement of grace, not just an occasional good feeling that may come along.

Contemplation has so much to offer us. It becomes our strong foundation in God and makes it possible for us to live with paradox and the unfolding mystery of God's presence and interaction with us. This is clearly not the way of our world with so many of its empty promises. Instead, it is a movement to wisdom and love. Richard Rohr defines it well, "Contemplation is meeting as much reality as you can handle without filters, judgments, or commentaries."[64] Actions of the heart are always tranquil, passive more than active, surrendering all the resisting, evaluating, and judging that occupy so much of my mind. All of these are turned over to the presence, and we are able to meet God on God's terms, not on our own. Then we encounter the goal of the psalmist's deepest longing: "My soul thirsts for God, for the living God. When shall I come and behold the face of God?" and Jesus as "The way, the truth, and the life."[65]

It is important to note that many contemplate without naming it as such for it can be done sitting in a boat fishing, gazing at a garden of flowers, mesmerized by the flutter of a butterfly, or sitting on a porch rocking.

---

[64] Adapted from Richard Rohr, *Yes, And…: Daily Meditations*, (Cincinnati: Franciscan Media, 2013), 407, 398.

[65] Psalm 42:2, John 14:6, (Revised Standard Version).

A THUMBNAIL HISTORY OF CONTEMPLATION

For our purposes, suffice it to say that contemplation is an integral part of our Christian tradition of prayer. I have dealt with this in greater detail in a prior work.[66] Did not Jesus engage in contemplative prayer prior to making every important decision? The Gospels speak of his going off by himself to be in the presence of the Father. Such moments were experiences of the heart, of union, of the deepest "resting in," and he always came out of them renewed, refreshed, and resolute, whether it was to be baptized and begin his ministry, choosing his apostles, going up to Jerusalem to meet the end of his earthly existence, or seeking the strength to endure his impending passion. While not the joy we would normally think of from such experiences, Jesus' resulting demeanor did speak of a quiet inner strength, a sense of fullness or satisfaction that could be considered a quieter, gentler side of joy.

From Jesus' practice, we move to the post Apostolic Age and Jesus' earliest of followers, who chose to live as hermits in the deserts of Syria, Palestine, and North Africa. In the 3rd Century, these desert mothers and fathers began to come together in coenobiums (monks coming together and stressing community rather than asceticism). They did so in order to celebrate the Eucharist. Father Anthony, among others, began to gather their living styles and customs, and in the 6th Century, they were put into a rule by St. Benedict of Nursia. From there, we might fast forward to the 12th Century and the reform of the monastery of Citeaux out of which came the name *Cistercian* by which the monks were called. Fast forward again to the 17th Century for still another reform from the Cistercian Abbey of La Trappe, from which came the earliest monks to America, now known as Trappists. Later in this chapter, we shall see how the Trappists took up the baton for contemplative practice in the last 50 years, but first, a bit about the foundational documents that underpin contemplative prayer.

FOUNDATIONAL DOCUMENTS FOR CONTEMPLATIVE PRAYER

There are, in the Christian Tradition, documents that ground and create the bedrock for contemplative prayer. Most notable among them is the *Philokalia, The Cloud of Unknowing* and the writings of Teresa of Ávila and John of the Cross. A word about each will help ground our understanding of contemplative prayer.

---

[66] Nicholas Amato, *Living in God: Contemplative Prayer and Contemplative Action*, (Bloomington: WestBow Press, 2016), 11-15.

The *Philokalia* is a work of Orthodox Christianity, written as a collection of sacred texts between the 4ᵗʰ and 5ᵗʰ centuries. It was the compilation of two Orthodox monks from two different monasteries, Nikodimos of Athos and Makarios of Corinth both in the 18ᵗʰ Century.[67] The compilation includes such early contemplatives as St. Isaiah the Solitary and his work *On Guarding the Intellect*, Evagrius, the solitary's *Outline Teaching on Asceticism and Stillness in the Solitary Life* and John Cassian's *On the Eight Vices*. Each work deals with different components of contemplative practice or what needs to be attended to for the greatest disposition of the one seeking God's presence.

The *Cloud of Unknowing* is an anonymous work[68] written in Middle English in the second half of the 14ᵗʰ Century.[69] It presents contemplative prayer as it was being practiced in the Middle Ages with an emphasis on knowing God and the abandonment of all thoughts of God's attributes and activities. What is required is the abandonment of all thinking and of the ego in order to enter into the mystery of "unknowing," where one is able to experience God as God is, without adding anything by way of image, ego, or mental considerations. The work speaks of thus coming to know the very nature of God. It must be remembered that this "knowing" is not mental comprehension or understanding, but more a habit of the heart that deals with surrendering in trust and love to the Beloved who awaits us in the silence. It is the passionate love of the union of lover and beloved that the writer of *The Cloud* had in mind when he wrote, "God can be held fast and loved by means of love, but by thought never."[70] "Love" is this author's pet word for that open, diffuse awareness, which gradually allows another and a deeper way of knowing to pervade one's entire being.

Teresa of Ávila and John of the Cross were both Carmelite mystics of the 16ᵗʰ Century. Teresa, as a Doctor of the Catholic Church, was a theologian for Mental Prayer. She developed a lexicon for the three kinds of prayer — verbal/vocal, meditation, and contemplation — and in her published works went into detailed descriptions of each. She was an important force in the Catholic Counter Reformation when the Reformers were confiscating monasteries, and contemplative prayer was falling into disuse. John of the Cross (1542-1591), along with Teresa of Ávila (1515-1582), was a founder of the reformed or discalced (not wearing shoes; going barefoot or in sandals)

[67] Andrew Louth, *Modern Orthodox Thinkers: From the Philokalia to the Present*, (Downers Grove: Intervarsity Press, 2015), 1. For a complete text of the Philokalia see: *The Philokalia, Volume 4: The Complete Text; Compiled by St. Nikodimos of the Holy Mountain & St. Markarios of Corinth* translated by G.E.H. Palmer, Sherrard, Kallistos and Ware, (London: Faber and Faber, 1999).

[68] The author is unknown. The English Augustinian mystic Walter Hilton has been suggested. Some claim the author was a Carthusian priest.

[69] Unknown Mystic, *The Cloud of Unknowing*, (New Kensington: Whitaker House, 2014).

[70] *The Cloud of Unknowing*, introductory commentary and translation by Ira Progoff translated by Ira Progroff, (New York: Delta Books, 1957), 72.

Carmelites. He was declared a Doctor of Mystical Theology by Pope Pius XI in 1926. Central to John's teaching was that the individual must empty himself of self in order to be filled by and united with God. True to this maxim, John assures his reader that as you move forward to this unitive state, more of your sins and shortcomings are disclosed to you. As these are removed, the individual enters into what he famously has called the "Dark Night," which is characterized as a passive cleansing of the soul or spirit. It is a time of great trials, but they are trials that are purgative or cleansing of the person's spirit. While the individual may have begun the process, it is God who is doing the cleansing. While it is passive, it is not inert, and the individual can indeed submit to the divine intervention. This purgation leaves the seeker free to act with a new sense of energy. This is the same greatness that is achieved by so many mystics. The individual emerges from the "Dark Night" into the full noonday sun, which John has described in *The Spiritual Canticle* and the *Living Flame of Love*. Here, in perfect contemplation, one's spirit becomes united to the divine nature. Here, the individual comes to understand the pain of the journey inward, as the joy of the glory now being revealed is received.[71] His major contributions to contemplative prayer include:

- ➤ *The Ascent of Mount Carmel,* where the journey begins, as John would say, "In a dark night with anxious *love* inflamed."

- ➤ *The Dark Night of the Soul* — This and the preceding work were written soon after his escape from nine months in *prison*, and, though incomplete, supplement each other, forming a full treatise on Mystical Theology.

- ➤ *Spiritual Canticle* is his work that is a paraphrase of the Old Testament's The Canticle of Canticles. It was begun during his *imprisonment* by his own friars and completed years later.

- ➤ John's poems and spiritual maxims complete his written contribution to contemplative prayer.

So contemplative prayer, we see from history, is nothing new. It is grounded in both practice and documents, sustained in monastic settings, and developed over the centuries. What a rich and valuable way to pray and encounter the Living God!

---

[71] Benedict Zimmerman, "*St. John of the Cross,*" New Advent, accessed January 18, 2017, http://www.newadvent.org/cathen/08480a.htm.

TERESA OF ÁVILA'S CONTRIBUTION AS THE GOLD STANDARD

In addition to developing the three kinds of prayer we discussed earlier, Teresa has spoken most poignantly about how contemplation is experienced. It can be experienced in one of three ways. The ways are developmental in that each grows out of the prior state. Each state is not experienced as a particular state in the moment but is clarified and understood upon reflection of what the time in prayer was like. She calls the states of contemplation: the Prayer of Recollection, the Prayer of Quiet, and the Prayer of Union.[72]

She speaks of the Prayer of Recollection in this way. When we make the effort to set aside time to be still and turn inward, we gather all our faculties to a single point of concentration and invite the presence of the sacred to enter us. In this state, we may find that what the Buddhists call "monkey mind" continues to chatter for a while, but gradually things settle down and a kind of spaciousness begins to open between the thoughts, and this is where the Holy One slips in to sit beside us. The Prayer of Recollection involves our active participation. It requires discipline, concentration, and a willingness to endure both mental turmoil and spiritual aridity. It is an act of purification; by scouring the vessel of our souls with the practice of prayer, we empty ourselves so that the Beloved may fill us.

At this point in the Prayer of Recollection, she speaks of entering the Prayer of Quiet. Now that the labor of recollection has cleansed us, we are ready to receive the infusion of divine light. This is a state of grace and is God's work. Once we have gathered our senses and intellect, a feeling of deep peace and quietude may wash over us like a warm wave. This is an exceedingly delicate experience. We cannot manufacture or manipulate this stage of prayer. We can only make ourselves ready to receive it when it comes and, in the words of the late meditation teacher Stephen Levine, we "hold on tightly and let go lightly."[73]

In Teresa's final stage, the Prayer of Union, any sense of an individualized self simply slips away. The soul merges with the divine, like a drop of water dropping into the boundless sea. The Beloved, who, as it turns out, has longed for the lover as fervently as she has desired him, makes her one with him. The Prayer of Union is usually fleeting, but its impact endures, so intense is the grace. Each time God blesses us with these unitive

---

[72] For a lengthier discussion of these, see: Jordan Aumann, O.P., "St. Teresa's Teaching on the Grades of Prayer," Catholic Culture, accessed January 18, 2017, www.catholicculture.org/culture/library/view.cfm?id=7725.

[73] Richard Rohr, "Spirituality of Imperfection: Week 2 Summary: Sunday, July 24–Friday, July 29, 2016," *Richard Rohr's Daily Meditation*, July 30, 2016, accessed January 19, 2017, https://cac.org/spirituality-imperfection-week-2-summary-2016-07-30/.

experiences, we are forever transformed. We are likely to still bumble through the human condition, behaving unskillfully at times and with more grace at others, but, with each taste of union, we identify a little less with our individual personality and more with our essential unity with the Divine. We are less likely to take passing circumstances as seriously as we used to. Our values shift from acquiring security to serving the One through our being of service in the world. The contemplative life is not a matter of achieving some artificial state of perfection available only to the spiritual elite. Teresa of Ávila is one of the great advocates and models of the power of simply sitting for a few minutes each day in silence and stillness, striking up a conversation with the One who is waiting to love us unconditionally, the One who will never leave us, the One who is not different from the essence of who we truly are.

THREE CISTERCIAN FOUNDERS

It was in the early 1960's, that Thomas Merton was writing books that called for a rediscovery of contemplative prayer. His call to rediscovery extended not only within the monastic enclosure, but also to all in all walks of life. It was Thomas Keating and John Main who responded to Merton's prophetic call. They set about developing easy to learn, easy to apply methods for meditation, which were rooted in the Christian spiritual tradition. A world hungry for a reconnection to its Christian roots was waiting. The new practices were not to be a graft onto Eastern meditation, nor were they to be trendy unrelated techniques that would quickly pass out of vogue. Instead, the practices needed to tap the very presence of God in our lives and to satisfy our deepest hungers for divine union.

I have had an interesting relationship with Centering Prayer. When Abbot Thomas Keating, William Meninger, and Basil Pennington were beginning to think of ways to make contemplative prayer more accessible to Catholics and people of all faiths, I was visiting their monastery of St. Joseph's Abbey in Spencer, Massachusetts from my seminary in nearby Connecticut. It was then, and continues to this day to be, a stunning setting for prayer and meditation. Several factors were coming together to create a rich dialogue around contemplation and how traditional practices might be rethought for contemporary seekers of this form of prayer.

Vatican II had declared that all Christians were called to holiness, and the Council encouraged Christians to interact with other traditions so as to enrich one another. The area of Spencer, Massachusetts was rich with retreat centers of both Eastern and Western practices. Prior to Vatican II, many Christians were leaving their churches behind for Eastern practices of prayer and for the Transcendental Meditation Movement. The goal behind the three

Trappists at St. Joseph's Abbey was to present the contemplative traditions in a more accessible manner, particularly to Christians, as a direct response to this call of Vatican II.

What these three monks did was to take the centuries' old tradition of contemplative prayer and distill it to a simpler formula that could be easily learned, remembered, and practiced by people in all walks of life. What in the end emerged has come to be known as Centering Prayer. The name itself was suggested by another Trappist monk, Thomas Merton, who described it as, "Centered entirely on the presence of God and His will and love, and as rising up out of the center of nothingness and silence."[74] Who would have guessed how popular the movement would become just fifty years after its inception, offering people grounding, transformation, and healing from an intimate union with God!

It was William Meninger who brought to the other two founders the idea of entering into a quiet state of communion with God. The idea was based on the 14th Century classic on contemplative prayer called *The Cloud of Unknowing,* and Meninger contributed the idea of using a single sacred word repeated as many times as necessary. It was a minimalist way of clearing the mind of all concepts and then simply letting go of the word. Once the practice was systematized, it was shared in retreats, initially given at St. Joseph's, but the demand outstripped the facilities, and Meninger and Pennington began training others to offer the retreats on Centering Prayer in other facilities. From there, Keating joined with emerging leaders of the practice and began organizing small faith communities that he called *Contemplative Outreach.* He also began a series of theological talks that were important in grounding centering prayer in solid theology, faithful tradition, and good psychology.

Thomas Keating continues to this day as the leading voice of the Centering Prayer movement and reminding his readers that Centering Prayer is not done with attention but with *intention.* There is no object or phrase for meditation. Keating wants us to see the sacred word as merely a minimal tool to move us from thinking of what it means in itself to it simply being a springboard, as is the breathing in and breathing out, as is the synchronization of the breathing and the word, as is the letting go. What is most important about the word is that it be your intention *both* to be with God and to live out of that presence. Returning to the word each time a thought enters your mind is a gentle way to return to your *intention, which* is what the word stands for.

After sitting in silence, it is reflecting on the word again and the experience in the silence that the individual may think of an action that flows from either the word or the experience that is initiated. Most often, my intention is to be totally open to God. I'll often use the motto of John Paul

[74] Joseph G. Sandman, *Centering Prayer: A Treasure for the Soul,* September 9, 2000, America, accessed January 20, 2017, http://www.americamagazine.org/issue/379/article/centering-prayer.

II, *Totus Tuus,* "All yours." Jesus assured his followers that what is going on in this prayer "in secret" is hidden even from the one praying, and that it is going on in that innermost room within us where our life is "Hid [Hidden] with Christ in God."[75] Whereas the *sacred word* in Centering Prayer serves as a placeholder for your intention, I believe, contrary to Keating and Bourgeault, that it can also serve as a mantra, which is repeated in synchronization to your breath, thus serving as an important tool to dispose you to a deep awareness.[76]

CONTRIBUTION OF JOHN MAIN

John Main[77] was a British Benedictine monk and Catholic priest who taught meditation and contemplative prayer using a mantra. He learned the technique from his working in Kuala Lumpur, Malaya, where he served in the British Colonial Service before becoming a monk. So moved was he by the practice that he began Christian meditation groups out of his monastery in West London and after that in Montreal, Canada. These have grown into what is today the *World Community for Christian Meditation.*

It was 1970, just after the Vatican Council and the ferment at St. Joseph's Abbey in Spencer, Massachusetts, that Main was assigned as Headmaster of St. Anselm's Abbey School in Washington, D.C. What he was able to do was connect the teachings of the desert father, John Cassian, to the meditative practices he had learned in Kuala Lumpur. His practice follows very closely the teachings of Keating regarding Centering Prayer.

> ➤ Sit still and upright
>
> ➤ Close your eyes lightly
>
> ➤ Sit relaxed and alert
>
> ➤ Begin to silently repeat a single word. He recommends *Maranatha* (Come, Lord Jesus)
>
> ➤ Repeat it as four syllables
>
> ➤ Do not imagine anything
>
> ➤ When distractions come, simply return to the word
>
> ➤ Repeat the practice 20-30 minutes each morning and evening

---

[75] Colossians 3:2-4 in context reads: "Set your minds on things that are above, not on things that are on earth. For you have died, and your life is hid [sic] with Christ in God. When Christ who is our life appears, then you also will appear with him in glory," (Revised Standard Version).

[76] Adapted from Cynthia Bourgeault, *The Heart of Centering Prayer: Nondual Christianity in Theory and Practice,* (Boulder: Shambhala, 2016), 17-20.

[77] "Everything you need to know about how to meditate in 128 words," accessed January 21, 2017, www.johnmain.org.

It would be interesting to know what correspondence, if any, there was between Keating and Main. Both were Benedictines (Trappists/ Cistercians are reformed Benedictines), both were influenced by Eastern mysticism, and both espoused the exact same teaching on contemplation, although Main referred to it as meditation and Keating, as contemplation.

THE CALL OF THE DEEP

What is this space of contemplation that satisfies so deeply? What is this thirst that is longing to be slaked? So many of the Psalms speak eloquently of our human experiences of thirst and satisfaction. This all too human longing arises deep within the heart of the psalmist as well, and its satisfaction is addressed honestly and poignantly to God. There is no hesitation from the psalmist to cry out, to challenge God's goodness, or to test God's patience. The 42nd Psalm is such an example. The imagery is beautiful and the feelings expressed, deeply human. Even if there were no God, as for the case of someone who doesn't believe, the most ardent non-believer would be able to identify with the pain and the longing, at least on a psychological level of one who does believe. One would think that that would, of its very self, open the person for God to manifest God's self in a way that would touch individuals wherever they find themselves.

I invite you to read the following excerpt of the Psalm, and then rest with it for a while in silence to see what it becomes for you.

As the deer longs for streams of water,

so my soul longs for you, O God.

My soul thirsts for God, the living God.

When can I enter and see the face of God?

…

Deep calls to deep

in the roar of your torrents,

and all your waves and breakers

sweep over me.

By day may the Lord send his mercy,

and by night may his righteousness be with me!

I will pray to the God of my life,

I will say to God, my rock:

"Why do you forget me?"[78]

---

[78] Psalms 42: 1-3, 8-10, (New American Bible (Revised Edition)).

The desert mothers and fathers of the Church knew of this thirst and the depths that satisfied it. Their earliest contribution to contemplative prayer was not to associate consciousness with the thinking mind. It was something more. Thomas Aquinas knew it as something more as well. He called it "connatural intelligence," claiming that it was true to one's own human nature and true to a larger nature as well. The American philosopher Ralph Waldo Emerson called consciousness, the "Over-Soul." In all cases, it is clear that through contemplation we plug into a consciousness that is larger than the thinking brain. It is experienced by a surrender to what is going on in my mind, and, in doing so, all the clutter is eliminated, and only the present moment remains. It is then possible to see things from a grander vantage point, without my limiting, self-centering ego getting in the way. And with such seeing comes a sense of humility, gratitude, and joy.

Knowing from consciousness is a different kind of knowing than a rational knowing, which is argumentative and involves analysis, reasoning, and judgments. No, consciousness brings forth quietude, compassion, and a knowing without any force of the intellect. We know deeply and assuredly. I am sharing in the life and viewpoint of the holy. In the constancy of committing ourselves to the great silence, we can acquire the habit of this constancy and increase the frequency of having God break through to us. Of this consciousness, Richard Rohr states,

> "Deep consciousness knows the true value of a thing, it knows intuitively what is real and what's unreal, what is eternal and what is passing, what matters and what doesn't matter at all. *This kind of consciousness allows us to see the archetypal truth within the particular,* [emphasis is Rohr's] for example the pattern of Christ's death and resurrection within each death and birth. At a loved one's deathbed we can be present to their dying, our dying, all dying — and to the reality of life changing forms in each death. If we can stay within this kind of consciousness, I can promise we'll receive compassion and empathy for the world. *In the big consciousness, we know things by participation with them, which is love.*[79]

The union that results is that the lover becomes one with the beloved. We live in God, and God lives in us. Thus, when I pray, it is God *already* praying in me. When I worship, it is God *already* worshipping in me. When I love, the same is true.

---

[79] Richard Rohr, *Everything Belongs: The Gift of Contemplative Prayer,* (New York: The Crossroad Publishing Company, 1999), 90-91.

GOING IN:
ATTENTION VERSUS INTENTION

"Pay attention!" is an all too familiar command to us to focus on a particular thing. In actuality, when we pay attention to something, we connect our thinking to an object out there — so there is a subject thinking and an object to which we are paying attention. Spiritual writers speak of a second kind of attention, where there is not this object and subject link, but a subject self-contained and aware, not linked to the awareness, of a thing or object. Rumi, the Sufi mystic, uses the analogy of mercury, when released on a flat surface, can either pool out as a puddle or retain itself like a ball. There is, in the latter, a tension that keeps it contained as a ball without it flowing out into a pool. Awareness, states Borgeault, is like that, "In its 'liquid' form, it connects subject to object. In its solid...form, it is a...field of vibratory awareness, within which you can be conscious of the whole without having to split the field into the usual subject/object polarity."[80] Tibetan Buddhists call this state *rigpa* or pure awareness and it is held to be a higher state of awareness, that reaches the innermost nature of the mind. This is our ultimate nature.[81]

In our Western tradition, we speak of remaining recollected, that is, not necessarily having thoughts, but being attentive or paying attention to each present moment as it is, without anything added on our part. It is not a willful teeth gritting effort to remain attentive, but a gentle presence to what is before you with a sense that all is well, no matter what the level of turmoil. You are "collected again;" you are re-collected in these moments. Employing this re-collected-ness, you are in touch with a deeper energy that brings forth a new and more powerful way of perceiving. It is like the drop of mercury Rumi speaks of that maintains its tension without puddling into objects. It is the state in which one's spirit finds itself, as Teresa of Ávila would say, in a "Well of limpid water, from which flow only streams of clearest crystal. Its works are pleasing both to God and man, rising from the River of Life, beside which it is rooted like a tree."[82]

---

[80] Bourgeault, Op. cit., 129–130, 134.
[81] "What is Rigpa," Rigpa, accessed January 28, 2017, http://usa.rigpa.org/about/#_rigpa.
[82] "Saint Teresa of Avila Quotes," Brainy Quote, accessed January 28, 2017, www.brainyquote.com/quotes/quotes/s/saintteres586987.html.

WHAT GOES ON IN THE "SPACE" OF "NO-SPACE"?

To speak of the state of contemplation as a place of no-space is not just playing with words. True, it is not a space, as a place in which some object is located. It is a space however, in the sense that one can be spiritually situated. And here is the important distinction, the "being situated" is unitive, that is, it is an experience of oneness with a reality that is boundlessly greater than oneself. Furthermore, in the moment, it may be experienced as that boundless reality or, after the prayer has ended, it may be experienced in the recollection of the time span that has now passed. In such a case, what is called forth or recalled is the joy of that union. To get to this union, one goes through different stages, which our tradition has called purgative, illuminative, and unitive.[83] Notice in the steps the movement forward from purgative stress to unitive joy. Yes, the joy is the experience of the unitive state. It is the overflowing into the emotions that the one praying experiences. It is the fruit, the result. It is how the presence is reflected in the person's emotions. In the unitive state, the ego has dissolved, and there is a shift in how the person views himself. What flows forth in this joy is a capacity to live beyond the narrower confines of self and self-interest. The oneness experienced with God creates the joy, and the joy serves to empower having a oneness with all we meet. This is not so much an act of willpower — the way we might build a muscle through willful weight training. It is more of a new way of seeing, understanding, and acting as oneself. It is a new sense of *being* that makes possible a new sense of *doing*. In the East, this union is more *monistic*. Monism holds that reality is only one unitary organic whole with no independent parts.[84] One's deepest identity, therefore, is a unity with all that is. Western thought sees this oneness or unity as essentially relational. It is to be fully one with the divine in likeness and relationship without being God. It is the union of the lover and the beloved, as the marriage rite attests where the Nuptial Blessing prays that the man and woman, "might be no longer two, but one flesh" and that, "what God was pleased to make one must never be divided."[85] Like the mystery of oneness in the Godhead, yet like the distinction in the Trinity of three persons, there is this same mystery lived in the contemplative presence between the one who prays and the Spirit. Paul, in addressing the Romans, attests that, "The Spirit itself bears witness with our spirit that we are children

---

[83] Reginald Garrigou-Lagrange, "The Three Ages of the Spiritual Life According to the Fathers and the Great Spiritual Writers," The Three Ages of the Interior Life, accessed January 28, 2017, http://www.christianperfection.info/tta26.php.

[84] *Merriam Webster Dictionary,* s.v. "monoism," accessed January 28, 2017, http://www.merriam-webster.com.

[85] "Nuptial Blessing from the Catholic Marriage Ritual," For Your Marriage, accessed January 28, 2017, http://www.foryourmarriage.org/the-nuptial-blessing/.

of God."[86] In another place he affirms, "All of us, gazing with unveiled face on the glory of the Lord, are being transformed into the same image from glory to glory, as from the Lord who is the Spirit."[87] These revelations within sacred scripture are clearly validated in the union experienced in contemplative prayer and reinforced with the human understanding we have of the love of marriage and friendship. In all these spheres of human-divine activity, the essential religious experience is that you find yourself being *known through.* It is a greater knowing than knowing something about yourself, having considerations of your own worthiness, or the need for merit.[88]

My own mother comes to mind as my earliest experience of being known through and through, so much so, that as a child and teenager, she was able to predict with a high degree of certainty what mischief or predicament I was about to get into. This experience of unconditional love that knows and still loves came home to me recently in a poem by Wendell Berry entitled: "To My Mother."

> I was your rebellious son,
>
> do you remember? Sometimes
>
> I wonder if you do remember,
>
> so complete has your forgiveness been.
>
> So complete has your forgiveness been
>
> I wonder sometimes if it did not
>
> precede my wrong, and I erred,
>
> safe found, within your love....[89]

Being in this sacred space is truly a different way of knowing. Being in this space removes our anxiety about having to figure it out with our reasoning and having to have someone give you an explanation beyond dispute. For the contemplative, God becomes more a verb than a noun, more a process than a conclusion, more an experience than a dogma, more a personal relationship than an idea. *The Prologue* of the Gospel of John assures us that Christ is a Living Word long before he was a written or spoken word:

> "In the beginning was the Word, and the Word was with God, and the Word was God. He was in the beginning with God; all things were made through him, and without him was not anything made that was made. In him was life, and the life was the light of men. The light shines in the darkness, and the darkness has not overcome it."[90]

---

[86] Romans 8:16, (New American Bible (Revised Edition)).
[87] 2 Corinthians 3:18, (New American Bible (Revised Edition)).
[88] 1 Corinthians 13:12, (New American Bible (Revised Edition)).
[89] Wendell Berry, *Entries*, "To My Mother," (Washington: Pantheon Books, 1994).
[90] John 1:1-5, (Revised Standard Version).

While nouns, conclusions, dogma, and ideas are safe and can be held without much personal engagement, we know that verbs, processes, experiences, and personal relationships are much more engaging, more mysterious, and possibly less capable of control on our part. And to imagine this happening between us and God can be a bit frightening. How is one to go about fulfilling this great inner longing? How is one to pray? St. Paul responds succinctly to the Romans: "Likewise the Spirit helps us in our weakness; for we do not know how to pray as we ought, but the Spirit himself intercedes for us with sighs too deep for words.[91] It is a great consolation then, that the space of no-space need not be feared and that we can allow ourselves to be bowled over by a God who is already seeking us, long before it was an idea to ourselves.

WHAT COMES OUT OF THIS "SPACE" OF "NO-SPACE"?

Father Marshall Craver is a long-time friend and Episcopal priest with whom I have walked the contemplative path over many years. His personal experience has taught him that there are three gifts that the silence offers: Gratitude, Guidance, and Generosity.[92] The Gratitude is a feeling of deep appreciation for the gift of the present moment. It is a recognition that right here, right now, God is grounding, nurturing, and healing me. "Yes, right now. No, right now. That moment is gone, so right now…" Just acknowledging that grounding, nurturing, and healing in each moment, quickens both its reception and its appreciation. Guidance is more than a feeling for Craver. It is like a magnet to metal filings; the rings of filings around each end of the horseshoe-shaped magnet make clear a direction, a path, and an affinity for good works. If each filing is a decision point, then the Guidance is the clarity of when to say yes and when to say no. Once again, it is more than just the knowing, it is the knowing *plus* the empowerment of grace in order to act, grace moving me from my intellect to my will. Generosity is not simply my wanting to give fully and freely. It is in loving others in their brokenness and loving others in my prior aversion to them for whatever reason. And when this is carried out beyond intention to concrete action, I will find myself breaking the barriers that formerly defined or limited my reaching out. Anyone, in any situation is worthy of my love! Such a love I now have is as unearned or undeserved, but flows from God's loving me. To make this a more conscious experience and a daily one, Craver, each evening includes reviewing his day and noting how his contemplative presence from the morning has played out

---

[91] Romans 8:26, (Revised Standard Version).

[92] Marshall Craver, Faculty Member of the Shalem Institute, Washington, D.C., phone conversation, February 9, 2017.

specifically in terms of gratitude, guidance, and generosity during the day.[93] It becomes a self-perpetuating growth in love of God that gets expressed in love of neighbor.

GOING IN TO CONTEMPLATION; COMING OUT

Going to this space of no-space has to do with having the tools that enable me to assume an inner stance that offers the least resistance in order to be overtaken by God's grace. People in love know all too well that they cannot make the experience of oneness just happen. On both parts, it takes an assumption that this inner stance makes the grace of union possible and allows it to overflow in such a way that it blesses all aspects of living. Yes, they are more loving toward each other, and, much to their surprise, they will find themselves more loving toward others. Each morning and evening as I sit in silence for a half-hour, I find myself assuming almost a childlike stance of knowing I may have not met the mark in holiness, but can say, "Here I am Lord, known through and through and loved just as I am and that is who comes to you now." It is an inner childlike stance that offers little or no resistance to being overtaken by God. James Finley calls this, "the godly nature of myself just the way I am."[94]

MEDITATION IS NOT CONTEMPLATION

I have already stated above that meditation in the East is what we in the West would call contemplation.[95] To complicate things a bit more, John Main uses the word meditation in speaking of contemplative prayer as does James Finley, which we will see later in this chapter. I prefer to use the three categories that Teresa of Ávila made famous, namely, verbal/vocal prayer, meditation, and contemplation and keep each distinct, since each relates differently to thinking and awareness. See Figure 1. Once we understand what we mean by each, and after we have considered the sources for each, we can see how contemplative prayer is a direct experience of the divine, whereas the divine presence in the other two is mediated through words, images, and created things. Without overstating it, it can be said that in contemplative prayer, we see God "face to face" without any limitations of our own seeing or our lack of creative imagination.

---

[93] This review of Craver's is part of a formal daily review called the Jesuit "examen."
[94] Adapted from James Finley, exclusive Center for Action and Contemplation, *Living School Curriculum*, Unit 1.
[95] See page 40.

Level of Prayer	Cognitive Activity	Sources	Characteristics or God's Presence
Verbal/Vocal Prayer	Words, Thoughts	Psalms, Scripture, Hymns, Music, Poems, Rituals, Formalized Prayers	God's presence conveyed through images, impressions, feelings
Meditative Prayer	Thoughts	Gospel Stories, Guided Meditations, Viewing Nature or Art	God's presence conveyed through images, impressions, feelings
Contemplative Prayer	Awareness	Sacred Word, Mantra, Breathing, Letting Go	God's presence is experienced directly and is unitive and in the moment is beyond words or images

Figure 6 Teresa's Three Levels of Prayer

Looking at Figure 6, this does not mean that verbal/vocal prayer (row 1) could not give rise to a word or words to then use as a mantra or Sacred Word for contemplative prayer (row 3). In doing so, we would, in effect, be switching from row 1 to row 3, and going deeper in our prayer. In a similar way, meditative prayer around a scene from the Gospel (row 2) could stir us so that a word bubbles up to the surface, and it could be used as a mantra or Sacred Word in contemplation. In this case row 2, meditation was a resource for row 3, contemplation.

IF CONTEMPLATION ISN'T FOR YOU

Many retreatants will often say they simply are not able to sit still in the silence without interruptive thoughts or an environment free of noise and lots of activity. What are they to do? After many attempts, it may be time to admit that contemplative prayer may not be for them.

They could be encouraged to try more meditative prayer, using bible accounts or meditation books, or audio clips of guided meditations. Instead of moving from meditation to contemplation with the help of a mantra, stay within the meditation and its rich imagery and put yourself squarely in the middle of the scene. Think "five senses" and imagine what you hear, see, smell, taste, and touch in the scene. If it is the Last Supper, describe what the food tastes like, the smell of oil lamps, and the warmth of the evening. Imagine Jesus looking at you the way he's looking at John the Beloved. Receive the cup from the Lord and taste the rich red wine, and so on. The opportunity for a contemplative connection may come when you imagine what Jesus is saying to you about your life and its stresses. How's he encouraging you now that he is leaving you? What's he asking of you personally in dealing with the stressful situation or the stressful people at work or at home? After such a meditation, you might enter your thoughts in a journal and see how they influence the rest of your day or, if you are meditating in the evening, how they may impact your sleeping.

However, even meditative prayer may not be for you. You may enjoy or are committed to praying the Liturgy of the Hours,[96] reciting the rosary, attending daily Mass, or using special devotions. The difference between verbal/vocal and meditative prayer is not that one uses words and the other does not. The difference is that verbal/vocal prayer uses *preset words* or a *preset formula* of words. Meditative prayer is not tied to any set formula of words but is more of a free flowing interaction and conversation with God. One writer has said that in verbal/vocal prayer, our aim is to mean what we say. In contrast, in meditative prayer, our aim is to say what we mean. So in verbal/vocal prayer, we are using the words of someone else, or in the case of the Lord's Prayer, the words of Jesus himself. They are preset for us. What is important here is that we stay focused and make sure that we really mean in our hearts what we are saying. The spiritual life will always require some verbal/vocal prayer. In fact, it is always essential and foundational to assure us that we do not overlook important aspects of our relationship with God. This is why the Church makes painstaking efforts in carefully proscribing "official" prayers of the Mass. Thus, these are preset verbal/vocal prayers. Collectively, they are supposed to express all of the important aspects of our relationship with God. Biblical prayers and prayers composed by saints or others are helpful in assuring that we focus on a particularly important aspect of God or the Lord. Verbal/vocal prayer is here to stay, and it can be very helpful to use when we are in stress, particularly if it is focused on that very challenge. The prayer of Teresa of Ávila is a great example in this regard:

> Let nothing disturb you,
>
> Let nothing frighten you,
>
> All things are passing;
>
> God only is changeless.
>
> Patience gains all things.
>
> Who has God wants nothing.
>
> God alone suffices.[97]

---

[96] Liturgy of the Hours (LOH) is the prayer of the Universal Church comprised of seven times of the day with specific prayers. Most who pray the LOH, pray Morning Prayer and Evening Prayer.

[97] "St. Teresa's Bookmark," Our Catholic Prayers, accessed January 30, 2017, http://www.ourcatholicprayers.com/st-teresas-bookmark.html.

What is primary is that we make sure that we *mean* what we say.[98] In the saying what we mean and the words of such prayer, and in the prayer being addressed to stress, overcoming obstacles, or having God as a stronghold, the grace of the prayer is able to break through and have an impact on our perception of the situation or give us the grace to persevere. It can open us to joy and a sense of hope.

PRAY AS YOU CAN, NOT AS YOU OUGHT

How well do we remember the "compare and contrast" essay questions from our high school days? How I dreaded them! Give me a True/False or multiple-choice test any day. As I look back on those days of sweat and nail biting, I now see why they were particularly challenging to me. You not only had to have the information for each of the things you were comparing or contrasting, but you also had to go through a fair amount of analysis of why one was better than the other, so it wasn't just remembering, it was putting your values, acuity, and ability to sound well-versed on the subject to the test.

As an adult, I came to realize how true the old adage "All comparisons are odious" was, and its truth lays in the fact that comparing could easily deny or minimize the value of the item we were comparing, or that, rather than appreciating its inherent goodness, we were looking for satisfaction beyond what was possessed in the here-and-now. In more recent years, I came upon the adage of spiritual writer James Martin, S.J. "Compare and despair,"[99] which spoke beautifully to the issue and, where comparing rather than appreciating what is present as it is, can lead to a dark end. Of course, this issue strikes at the heart of dualistic thinking captured in the forced choice of either/or. When we move instead from a both/and perspective and accept the diversity and hold the paradox, then the space within us opens up and "compare and contrast" are recognized for the limitations they have and can finally be put to rest. A both/and perspective, wherever you are with stress, joined with a contemplative prayer practice — or if your prayer form is verbal/vocal or meditative — can be used as a springboard to a higher unity for a more effective, long lasting relief and joy. The shift from dualistic thinking to unitive thinking is akin to moving from the head to the heart and from the heart holding the dichotomy with the grace that is contemplative prayer. Thus, the head/heart shift and the three forms of prayer become bridges or portals

---

[98] John Wright, S.J., *"Prayer,"* The New Dictionary of Catholic Spirituality, ed. Michael Downey, (Collegeville: The Liturgical Press, 1993), 773.

[99] James Martin, S.J., *The Jesuit Guide to (Almost) Everything: A Spirituality for Real Life,* (San Francisco: HarperOne, 2012), 381-385.

to moving from stress to joy and thus the title of the present work. This both/and is more than a preference for me. It has become a lifestyle that is hopeful, life giving, and transformational.

Rather than contrasting and comparing, what it comes down to is developing a familiarity with all three types of prayer and seeing them all as portals, facets, or pathways to a deeper experience of God's presence. Teresa of Ávila was credited with advising her sisters to, "Pray as you can, not as you ought." That advice has stood the test of time.

DIALECTICAL THINKING AND THE JOY OF CENTERING PRAYER

Dialectical thinking is a common method that the human brain uses to understand concepts of any kind. When you examine the opposite of something, your brain can understand the world and the people in it, so it is with hot/cold, love/hate, now/later. Dialectical thinking is an important part of developing empathy insofar as the person using dialectical thinking must consider each opposite extreme. He would be committed to look each time at both extremes of an issue.[100]

Richard Rohr holds that when you play the two off of one another and then come to a *tertium quid,* a third something, this moves things to a new level. In the wisdom of many religious, this is often called the "Third Force." Rohr continues, "It is the process of overcoming seeming opposites by uncovering a reconciling third that is bigger than both of the parts and doesn't exclude either of them."[101] So, it isn't either pain *or* joy, but it is more pain *and* joy and how the two reconcile into a third experience. This third reality is bigger than the sum of the two and does not exclude either. This reality moves you to a new level of experience.

Paul in his epistles uses either/or thinking when he speaks of either the flesh or the spirit, the law or freedom, male or female. And yet, while he holds both without eliminating either, he moves to a reconciling third, which is a large space filled with the grace and compassion of God — this he calls the "New Creation."[102] Notice, Paul is not speaking dialectically, as in it having to be either one or the other. It is the new third reality that is the New Creation.

Another way to look at this interaction of two extremes reconciling themselves into a third higher reality is to see this third reality as mediating or reconciling the two from which it came. So it is not about two extremes

---

[100] *"Examples of Reasoning,"* Reference, accessed January 30, 2017, www.reference.com.

[101] Richard Rohr, "The Third Way," Richard Rohr's Daily Meditation, August 26, 2016, accessed January 31, 2017, https://cac.org/the-third-way-2016-08-26/.

[102] *"For neither circumcision counts for anything, nor uncircumcision, but a new creation,"* Galatians 6:15, (Revised Standard Version).

balancing themselves out, but a third that is calling them forth. Cynthia Bourgeault asserts:

> "In contrast to a binary system, which finds stability in the balance of opposites, the ternary system stipulates a third force that emerges as the necessary mediation of these opposites and that in turn generates a synthesis at a whole new level. It is a dialectic whose resolution simultaneously creates a new realm of possibility."[103]

We will see how the two opposites — "stress and no stress" — when confronted, acknowledged and owned, and are brought into the silence, open to a higher third reality — God's grace — that becomes available to the individual, which becomes the source of lasting joy.

The stoning of the woman caught in adultery is a vivid biblical example.[104] To stone her or not to stone her is the issue. Jesus by his poignant statement, "Let anyone among you who is without sin be the first to throw a stone at her," [105] gives rise to the higher third reality — compassion. Clearly either/or is not the choice, but both/and gives rise to the new level of reality called compassion. To repeat, looking at it from the third level, compassion has a drawing power that reinforces the futility of either/or thinking and acting. It is sad, but no less true that most in our world of politics and economics operate under binary or either/or thinking. Contemplative prayer allows us to live with dichotomies and to know that one pole or its opposite need not be forcibly selected. In the presence of God, both can be held, and we can thus give God the space to deliver the joy, which reconciles the two opposites and heals the soul.[106] Contemplation, then, can be seen as a state that helps us loosen the shackles of dichotomous thinking, as well as being a drawing or motivational force, inspiring us to live a life of greater union with God and others.

EGO CONSCIOUSNESS AND CONTEMPLATION

James Finley, a psychologist and spiritual writer, defines ego consciousness as, "The self-reflective bodily self in time and space, which is our usual day-by-day consciousness. Ego manifests itself in saying, "I want, I think, I need, I feel, I remember, I like, I don't like."[107] He holds that there is aspects of

---

[103] Cynthia Bourgeault, *The Holy Trinity and the Law of Three*, (Boston: Shambhala, 2013), 16.

[104] John 8:3-11, (Revised Standard Version).

[105] John 8:7, (Revised Standard Version).

[106] Cynthia Bourgeault, *The Shape of God: Deepening the Mystery of the Trinity*, (Center for Action and Contemplation: 2005), disc 4, (CD, DVD, MP3 download).

[107] James Finley, *Christian Meditation: Experiencing the Presence of God*, (New York: HarperSanFrancisco, 2004), 1-3, 5-7.

this ego consciousness that can help me experience less stress and thus help me achieve a greater sense of calm in relationship to myself, as well as toward others. This consciousness that is all about me is very restrictive and confined and can never satisfy our deeper values for union and intimacy with others. We came forth from the womb with a longing that was implanted within us as are our appetites, where the only proper and satisfying object for them is God himself. Contemplative prayer provides us the opportunity of releasing ourselves from this ego consciousness and self-absorption to bask in a God-consciousness that is much vaster and incomparably more satisfying and joy producing.

TRUE SELF–FALSE SELF

Our true self was described by Thomas Merton as the deepest "who" we could be, our deepest identity. At this level, the self is united to God and mirrors God's love and God's grace. In contrast, the false self is caught up in ego preservation and ego identity, as in my identity is in my family's genes, my salary, my title, my car, etc. This is a self that is completely out of sync with God's presence and clearly reflects sin in many of its aspects and general ignorance of what is real. Ego consciousness will keep us from ever knowing our deeper selves.

For Merton, a fruitful spiritual life was ridding or dismantling our false self and so disposing us to experiencing our true self beneath. In his development of Centering Prayer on a more psychological base, Keating saw the false self as more systemic, that is, our false selves were acquired in our nurturing — each time our needs were not met at home, in school, or in our social groups. Centering Prayer becomes a bit of a "time out," when we can literally take a breath, speak a word that speaks of the sacred, and so relaxing ourselves that we can gently glide into another dimension of what is truly real and be nurtured there without the ego-centered values to which we have clung for so long.

GIFTS RECEIVED
FROM CONTEMPLATION

In addition to coming face-to-face with the divine and being enhanced by that union, the graces of that union begin to flow into the life of the believer. Those who practice Centering Prayer speak of those extraordinary benefits.[108] They include:

> ➤ Greater access to God's own wisdom and energy

> ➤ Significant increase in creativity

> ➤ Decrease in compulsive behavior

> ➤ Reduction of painful emotions and negative thoughts

> ➤ Greater freedom to respond positively to them when they do arise

> ➤ Greater ability to accept difficult situations with peace and joy

> ➤ Expanded capacity to accept others on their own terms without judging them or desiring them to change

> ➤ Ability to love others more selflessly

> ➤ Greater awareness of the presence of God in every person and situation we encounter.

THE FRUITS OF CONTEMPLATION

We experience the fruits of contemplative prayer in one of two ways. At each extreme of the continuum they might be something like, "What happened to Fred!" and "She prays and prays and nothing seems to change for her."

For starters, we want both to affirm that contemplative prayer does bear fruit and second, that those effects can be seen in the daily life of the person. We should not look for signs that our prayer is working *during* the time we are sitting in silence. Where to begin to look for them, instead, is how that silence impacts you. I have covered in detail in a previous work[109] how the reflecting on a word chosen and the experience of the silence both become the ground for an intention of how your prayer may make a

---

[108] Sandman, Op. cit.

[109] Nicholas Amato, *Living in God: Contemplative Prayer and Contemplative Action,* (Bloomington: WestBow Press, 2016), 69ff.

difference in your choices today. Cynthia Bourgeault speaks of the subtlest fruit of contemplative prayer as,

> "A gradually deepening capacity to abide in the state of attention of the heart…You might describe this as a stable state of mindfulness or 'witnessing presence,' but emanating from the heart, not the head, and thus free of intrusion from that heavy-handed mental 'inner observer.' Once you get the hang of it, attention of the heart allows you to be fully present to God, and at the same time fully present to the situation at hand."[110]

The situations at hand come to us by direct encounter, as in a misunderstanding between friends, or more globally, as the conflict and violence in the Middle East. No matter, we are now more present to all events, as they come to our attention. It is with an intention of our hearts that will make all the difference in how we engage these situations and move from them to a more loving compassionate stance. With such an understanding, we can readily see the important part that contemplation has to play in our own healing and transformation and for that of the world at large. Contemplation is not a luxury for the few, *but is open to all.* It can give structure to how we see things and a systematic way of being conscious and present, both of which open our hearts to compassion and care for one another.

EFFECTS OF MEDITATION AND CONTEMPLATION ON OUR DNA

The positive effects that meditation and contemplation have on stress reduction have been long known. What has not been known until recently is that such forms of stillness can actually reverse the molecular reactions in our DNA that are a cause of poor health and even depression. Research recently published in the journal, *Frontiers in Immunology*, covers more than ten years of studies (18 studies involving 846 participants over 11 years) that analyze how gene behavior is affected by meditation and contemplation.[111]

---

[110] Bourgeault, Op. cit., 36, 38–39.
[111] Coventry University, "Meditation and yoga can 'reverse' DNA reactions which cause stress, new study suggests," June 15, 2017, accessed June 18, 2017, https://www.sciencedaily.com/releases/2017/06/170615213301.htm.

When an individual is exposed to stressful events, the sympathetic nervous system creates a "fight-or-flight" response. At the same time, the production of a molecule called nuclear factor kappa B (NF-kB), which regulates how our genes are expressed, takes place. The study shows that individuals who meditate and contemplate have the very opposite effect, that is, there is actually a decrease in the NF-kB produced. This leads to a reversal of the pro-inflammatory expression of the gene pattern. It is the expression of NF-kB that raises the risk of diseases caused by inflammation. Ivana Buric, the lead investigator of the project from the Brain, Belief and Behavior Laboratory in Coventry University's Center for Psychology, Behavior and Achievement states:

> "Millions of people around the world already enjoy the health benefits of mind-body interventions like yoga or meditation, but what they perhaps don't realize is that these benefits begin at a molecular level and can change the way our genetic code goes about its business."[112]

Clearly, meditation and contemplation cause the brain to impact our DNA processes in ways that not only reduce our stress, but also improve our overall well-being at a foundational level.

EFFECT OF "LETTING GO" OF THOUGHTS

It appears that neuroscience and spirituality, respectively, shed light on each other as a discipline. When we let go of thoughts — I am thinking of Teresa of Ávila and Thomas Keating — a space is provided to the individual that they did not have before. Scientists tell us that neural wiring is changed. New paths in the brain are created or strengthened that make real the possibilities for new choices. Rather than releasing your thought and creating a space of emptiness to be filled by the divine, Bourgeault, states, "I prefer to come at it from a slightly different angle, gently but firmly insisting that one does not release a thought in order to achieve some desired result; the releasing itself is the full meaning of the prayer."[113] It relates a bit to St. Paul speaking to the Corinthians: "For who has known the mind of the Lord so as to instruct him?" But we have the mind of Christ."[114] Letting go of a thought is akin to Jesus' own position of letting go even of his divinity to

---

[112] Ivana Buric, Miguel Farias, Jonathan Jong, Christopher Mee, Inti A. Brazil, "What Is the Molecular Signature of Mind–Body Interventions? A Systematic Review of Gene Expression Changes Induced by Meditation and Related Practices," June 16, 2017, accessed June 18, 2017, *Frontiers in Immunology*, http://journal.frontiersin.org/article/10.3389/fimmu.2017.00670/full.

[113] Bourgeault, Op. cit., 36, 38-39.

[114] 1 Corinthians 2:16, (Revised Standard Version).

become fully human. In theology, this is referred to as "kenosis." This letting go with practice can become our modus vivendi, self-emptying continuously to all that would upset or disturb. It would be having the mind of Jesus in all our choices. The tiny miniscule space between the letting go of one thought and the creation of another becomes a moment of alertness and openness, a moment of awareness without an object of thought. It is in such moments that the divine presence can break through and be experienced as God is in Godself. Thus, moments such as this, as they increase in length and frequency, become the ground for a life that is truly lived in God and the joy of that union. And to think it all began with the simple practice of letting go of thoughts!

CHILDHOOD CAVEATS

Anyone who grew up in the 1960's or earlier will remember what came across loud and clear in our Catholic School, CCD classes, or at home about contemplation. Contemplation was often presented as a state too lofty to attain and certainly out-of-reach for us "ordinary people." I can remember where the slightest interest in contemplation was thought of as that greatest of all sins — spiritual pride! If I would continue to ask about it, I was met with the story of my great uncle, who long ago in Italy lost his mind trying to understand God. If that did not put a stop to the queries, the old familiar story, which was a lot less foreboding than losing your mind, was of the little boy who kept running from the seashore to his hole in the sand with a little pail, trying to put the ocean into the hole. It was used to explain how hopeless our little minds were in knowing God. I learned later, as an adult, that the story was St. Augustine's. Stories and cautions notwithstanding, the spontaneous spiritual experiences I was experiencing as a child and a youth, deeply satisfied an innate appetite and longing for the divine, the longing I had for a hidden core within my very being. An ant hill, a leaf floating down a stream, a piece of instrumental music — it did not take much — would find me dissolving into presence, of sinking into the present moment with awareness. Thankfully, they continued to grow in spite of the lack of understanding or support.

SECULAR AND RELIGIOUS MYSTICS

A mystic is defined as a person who seeks by contemplation and self-surrender to obtain unity with, or absorption into, the Deity or the absolute, or who believes in the spiritual apprehension of truths that are beyond the intellect.[115] It would seem that the acquiring of the habit of contemplative

---

[115] "Mystic," Online Google Dictionary, accessed February 3, 2017,
    http://google-dictionary.so8848.com.

prayer would put one into that category. From this union, one no longer needs reasoned answers for the mysteries that surround their very lives. Oh, they still use their reason at work, solving problems, or making a case within the family or their circles of friends. But for the mysteries of life, the bigger deeper questions of pain, suffering, love, death, and unexpected consequences, the mystic has a deeper well from which to drink. The self-surrender that has brought about their unity with the divine has made all the difference for how they are able to deal with stresses of daily living.

Most of us could name individuals both within established churches, those of other faiths, and even those with no faith at all, who seemed to be in touch with a higher power. So, it is very possible to speak of both religious mystics and secular mystics. I have a dear friend of many years who claims to be an atheist, though he was raised as a Christian. He spends great swaths of time each day in reflection and union with spiritual truths beyond what is seen. As the owner and operator of his own landscape company, he enjoys being out each day in nature cutting acres of grass, trimming long lengths of shrubbery, and pruning scores of trees. He is so in union with the spiritual in the work he does that it seems to pervade every aspect of his being.

Several months ago, this dear friend, whose name is John, was diagnosed with advanced Pancreatic cancer. Only the month before the diagnosis, we had been hiking together, and he had no symptoms whatsoever at the time. With the eventuality of death looming large, I began taking regular trips to see him, as he was going through horrendous amounts of deadly chemotherapy before they could operate, hopefully to remove parts of his pancreas. Never have I seen so serene an individual facing death. For him, his mysticism was not "surrendering to obtain unity with or absorption into the Deity or the absolute," but it was clearly and unmistakably the "spiritual apprehension of truths that are beyond the intellect." On my visits, we began sharing things in life that have expressed the deepest values we espouse.

One time when it was his turn, he chose to share the second movement of Mahler's *Resurrection Symphony,* and, after listening to it together, he spoke eloquently of how it expressed his deepest feelings about death. As I listened to it, my own experience was one of triumph over death, and more deeply, a sense of my own triumph over *my* final death. In reflection after, I could savor the victory, as won for me personally by the Lord Jesus. While John understood my connection to the resurrection of the Lord, he was not able to experience the feeling of that victory. His was more the victory of facing death nobly and with serenity.

Might we then speak of two types of mystics? A religious mystic and secular mystic? And because of where and how they experience transcendence, the secular mystic has no need to look beyond the symphony he is composing or the lawnmower he is driving in order to live out the vision experienced in the silence. Their daily choices are for the common good. They care for others and the needy. However, in John's case, it seems they feel no need for a community of like-minded believers to join. They are ready to go it alone. The religious mystic, on the other hand, experiences a personal relationship with the divine and moves with energy or grace out of that union to a shared experience with other believers within a faith community. To gather regularly for song, hearing the word, and praising that inner presence are very important to that individual. Clearly, we have a religious mystic in this regard.

MYSTICS OF MANY COLORS

I would thus conclude that we have many types of mystics. For the Christian Mystic, the source of Centering Prayer is the Trinity, experienced as the divine life within us. For him, the reality of this Divine Indwelling is the most important of all the principles of the spiritual life. Yes, God's very own life is communicated to us, although it is beyond our ordinary faculties to perceive or understand it. It takes faith to access this presence.[116] Then, there is the atheistic mystic, like John.[117] He is in touch with the spiritual foundation within himself, and it is communicated with creation in its many forms and expressions. Here, there does not seem to be the necessity for a communal presence of others, nor is there a need to worship. A third type is the individual who believes in God and relates to a group with creedal beliefs and a community of like-minded believers. One such group is the Center for Spiritual Living. Highlights of their creed include belief in:

> ➢ God, the Living Spirit Almighty — One, indestructible, absolute, and self-existent Cause.

> ➢ The incarnation of Spirit in everyone and that all people are incarnations of the One Spirit.

> ➢ The eternality, the immortality, and the continuity of the individual soul.

> ➢ That Heaven is within us and that we experience it to the degree that we become conscious of it.

> ➢ The unity of all life…that God is personal to all who feel this indwelling Presence.

[116] Thomas Keating, *Reflections on the Unknowable*, (Brooklyn: Lantern Books, 2014), 15.
[117] See page 74.

> The direct revelation of Truth through the intuitive and spiritual nature of the individual…

> The Universal Spirit, which is God, operates through a Universal Mind which is the Law of God and that we are surrounded by this Creative Mind which receives the direct impress of our thought and acts upon it.

> Our own soul, our own spirit, and our own destiny for we understand that the Life of all is God.[118]

Finally, I would be remiss if I did not include still another type of Mystic. This person wavers between being a religious and being a secular mystic. In my own pastoral care of Catholics and former Catholics, I encounter many who have left the Church and "gone East" to Zen Buddhism or other non-religious affiliated meditation groups. They could no longer accept all the dogmatic and biblical teachings of their church. When I encounter them in retreat ministry, I advise such folks of the longing within them for an intimacy that is deeper than the religion they are fleeing; it is a personal relationship with the divine. This they can grasp and affirm. It is on this bedrock of intimate union with God that a desire for communing with others becomes a deeply felt need. In ritualizing this desire and rooting it in a family of faith, religion finds its expression. The very word religion is thought to be from the Latin *religare* meaning to bind.[119] Contemplative prayer then can serve as the beginning of a journey into a church, temple or mosque, where you can continue to grow within a community. Some resources that I have found helpful to advise others to read include: *Living Buddha, Living Christ* by Thich Nhat Hahn, *Jesus, A Pilgrimage* by James Martin, and *Without Buddha I Could Not Be a Christian* by Paul F. Knitter.

JOY JOLTS:
CONTEMPLATIVE TIDBITS

It often happens that in the midst of a stressful day something will come up to jolt me with a feeling of joy. I can look and rest for a moment in a treasured photo of a loved one on my desk, or I might think and savor for a moment the dinner engagement I have for later this evening, or I call a friend and sink into a brief one-on-one sharing regarding something we both value. Such tidbits that help me turn down the faucet on the stress-producing cortisol that my brain is emitting and turn up the faucet of the

---

[118] "Our Beliefs," Center for Spiritual Living, accessed February 3, 2017, http://www.cslftlauderdale.org/our-beliefs/.

[119] *Merriam Webster Dictionary*, s.v. "religion," accessed February 3, 2017, http://www.merriam-webster.com.

pleasure-inducing compound, dopamine, in my pre-frontal cortex, can contribute a quick fix regarding stress. Though they may not last long or lead to a long-term solution to my stress, they are temporary aides that help me lay my stress aside and draw from a deeper well, using objects and persons in my world. A word of clarification regarding our being proactive for joy jolts. The photo, recalling the coming evening's dinner, or the phone call are mediums that dispose us to grace and gratitude. They do not force God to give us joy. They allow us an inner stance that offers little resistance so we can be overtaken by the grace as it were.

Such disclosing moments can also come spontaneously. Suddenly, your awareness of a particular "this thing" awakens you to a greater "that thing" which transcends *this*. I will very often have a repeated succession of such awakenings when I am hiking around a lake and through woodland near my home or browsing in a museum. I remember seeing Picasso's *Guernica* for the first time in the *Museo Nacional Centro de Arte Reina Sofía* in Madrid, Spain. I was not able to pull myself away from it. Not only its size, but its depicted horror of war took me to a place I had never been in feeling compassion and empathy for the innocent victims that violence creates.[120] Oftentimes, just strolling along a quiet path praying Evening Prayer will assure me of the fact that nothing is missing anywhere in my world at that moment. As Finley would say, "The reality of everything around us is manifesting the fullness of reality itself."[121] We do not really have to spend extended periods of time in stress. At those times, there are joy jolts available, either of our own creation or their occurring spontaneously by getting out and about. I am always amused at the contemplative states that folks walking dogs can experience as they stroll through their neighborhood. There is no need to go about stressed so much of your day. Think of such stressors as perfect moments for a joy jolt. There are more than these fleeing tidbits I am speaking about. They are merely the outer perimeter of a much deeper world of grace and presence that can be accessed for longer periods of time by developing a habit of contemplative prayer that, when lived out of, does not allow the stresses to arise. It is grace, as being received before the stress, rather than being stressed and turning oneself over to the Lord to be healed. The former is proactive, and the latter is reactive. Joy jolts, occurring spontaneously or intentionally sought, give us a ready remedy to dealing with the stresses of daily living.

---

[120] *Guernica* was painted by Cubist Spanish painter, Pablo Picasso, in 1937. Its title *Guernica* is named after the city that the Nazis bombed in the Spanish Civil War. It depicts the horrors of war.

[121] Finley, Op. cit., 43, 45-50, 65-66.

A PERSONAL JOURNEY
FROM STRESS TO JOY

My earliest experience of being able to move from stress to joy really begins with my young boyhood ability to sit in silence and simply reflect. It may have been lying in the grass watching an army of ants working industriously to build their anthill, or it may have been sitting by the stream watching a leaf carried by the flow over rocks and into eddies. I wasn't sure it was meditation or contemplative prayer in those days; it was more delighting in the mystery of nature. To that were added smells and scents of flowers and fresh air, then shades of green in trees' leaves as the late afternoon sun filtered through with light and shadows and a multitude of hues of green, or scents of sautéing onion or garlic from my mother's stove. When childhood stresses arose, I had a place to run — either real and in the moment or vicariously through a remembered scene, scent, or feeling. Who knew then that I was developing an informal system of being able to move from stress to joy? Eventually, I learned lots more about both sides of the reality: how to handle stress and how to dispose myself to a deeper presence. It was not until I understood how nature and grace interact and build on one another that the paradigm became more complete.

Such beauty and perfection sensitized me to the beauty present in things I enjoyed doing with and for other people. In my teenage years, it was stopping by on the way home from school and visiting with "old" people and sharing a cup of coffee, working hard and clearing underbrush for a neighbor, or talking to older subscribers on my paper route delivering *The Long Island Press*. There was a compassion that began to grow that recognized the preciousness of what seemed broken or misplaced in my little world, like wanting to dance with girls that were not asked to dance in a junior high mixer or talking to the boy from Estonia who was ignored because he was a "foreigner." One would think that being compassionate is borne of an intention to be so. I see now that it was more of a giving myself to the beauty I found in the silence and embracing the presence of God that was empowering me. It was as if God's compassion for me was flowing through me and opening or manifesting itself in what appeared as my own brokenness or the brokenness of others. I am reminded of the Prodigal Son[122] who appears in his brokenness to return and ask his father's forgiveness, yet is unable to even begin his practiced apology, before his loving father throws his arms around him, kisses him, showers him with gifts expressing honor and welcome, and throws him an extraordinary celebration. And all this without even a word of apology on his lips, but only the desire to return.

---

[122] Luke 15: 11-32, (Revised Standard Version).

MOVING IN A NEW DIRECTION

A review of the preceding chapters would see a shift or a movement forward on several fronts. I have built on the years of practice of contemplative prayer as it was developed by Thomas Keating. From my daily practice over the past 40 years and from teaching it on retreats for more than ten years, I have expanded the use of "sacred word," from where it can be drawn, teaching deep breathing, synchronizing the word to the breathing, and letting go to move one into awareness and the presence. A prior book of mine[123] goes into specific ways of dealing with distraction and intrusive thinking, as well as ways to reflect after the silence. From that reflection, we form different types of intentions that could be applied to choices as one's day evolves. Tracking those intentions and looking at the changes between intentions and actions that were finally done are helpful in discerning how God's grace is calling you forward.

In some, there are powerful resources supporting one's efforts and desire to enter the presence, and there are powerful resources supporting one's efforts at taking the grace received in contemplation and shaping it into concrete acts of compassion and kindness toward others. A reality that is experienced in doing so is that the actual actions become the realization of God moving through you to others. And, whether it is the overcoming of stress or compassion and love expressed toward the stressor, what is accomplished is "by God's grace" and our cooperation with and through that grace. In such ways, we recapture the joy within us.

As we move from Chapter 4 to Chapter 5, we find ourselves at a watershed for moving from stress to recovering our inner joy. My hope is that the present work, different from many in that it attempts to meld the psychology of outward stress to the spirituality of inner joy and connect the two with sound practices for doing so, will be a contribution to a more holistic way of dealing with stress and recapturing the joy within us. Let us then turn to a deeper understanding of stress, when it is good and when it is not, and effective ways to acknowledge it, manage it effectively, and have contemplative prayer assist us in both relieving it and capturing joy.

---

[123] Nicholas Amato, *Living in God: Contemplative Prayer and Contemplative Action*, (Bloomington: WestBow Press, 2016).

ANOTHER WORD ON NATURE AND GRACE

Let us return to the reality of nature and grace that we have already considered[124] as we draw this chapter to a close. Both we have said are really two sides of a single continuum. As such, each one impacts the other and the other impacts in return. As nature is unburdened by stress (psychology), the way is opened for grace to have a greater impact on the individual (spirituality). And the converse is just as true. As grace from prayer opens the person to self-acceptance and healing, the way to greater self-understanding opens. But the impact of each on the other is not just a back-and-forth movement. Think of it more as a staircase with each set of stairs — one nature, the other grace — having an impact that raises you to a higher level in the skyscraper. And surely you may find yourself going back down to a lower staircase because of a lapse in stress understanding or in an ineffective day or two at contemplative prayer, but you're still "in the building" and on a staircase and not in the basement, necessarily, but even there, you can always begin the climb again from either nature or grace.

MOVING FORWARD

I would suggest that we need to live with a sense of adventure even in the stress or dry periods of prayer in which we may find ourselves. We need to be explorers of a sort and with a hope that there is land beyond the horizon of the stormy sea. We continue looking at stress and practicing contemplative prayer with that hope in our hearts. Where we begin, either with a better understanding of the stress, or of the joy or reverie of silent presence, doesn't matter. It will take movement, and it will also take the silence of standing still emotionally, psychologically, and spiritually. T.S. Eliot summed it up well in his poem "East Coker."[125]

> Old men [sic] ought to be explorers
>
> Here and there does not matter
>
> *We must be still and still moving* [emphasis mine]
>
> Into another intensity
>
> For another union, a deeper communion

It is time to turn to acknowledging our stress, managing it, and taking it to the contemplative prayer that we have developed in this chapter.

---

[124] See page 6.

[125] T.S. Eliot, *"East Coker,"* accessed February 5, 2017, http://www.coldbacon.com/poems/fq.html.

Reflection Questions for Chapter 4: Contemplation

- *Jesus promises us "joy to the full." How realistic might the promise be for you?*

- *What keeps you from this "fullness of joy"?*

- *How would you describe your prayer life?*

Chapter 5:
Stress Relieving Techniques

Introductory Comments
1. Introduction
2. Summary of Handy Guides

Stress
3. Stress and Stressors; Positive & Negative Stress: What's the difference?
4. Levels of Stress and Initial Ways to Manage Them
5. Monday, Wednesday, and Friday's Child
6. Bringing the Ideas Home

Levels of Stress
7. Examples of High or Moderate Stress
8. Critical Stress Levels
9. Managing High Stress
10. Managing Moderate Stress
11. Managing for Joy
12. Can You Have "Unfelt" Joy?
13. Bringing the Ideas Home

Positive Aspects of Stress
14. Getting Stress to Work for You

Moving Forward
15. Where Is God in All This?
16. Stress Levels 5 and 3 as Portals to Contemplation and Resulting Joy
17. Movement Forward in the Literature

On the Cusp of Joy
18. Maintaining the Joy Within
19. Realization of Gospel Joy
20. Living the Day in Joy
21. Arriving at the Joy Within

INTRODUCTION

Let us lean on the words of Sirach, as we begin to reflect on techniques for relieving stress.

"Set your heart right and be steadfast,

and do not be hasty in time of calamity.

Cleave to him and do not depart...

Trust in him, and he will help you;

make your ways straight, and hope in him.

You who fear ["revere"] the Lord, trust in him,

and your reward will not fail;

you who fear the Lord, hope for good things,

for *everlasting joy* [emphasis added] and mercy.

Whoever trusted in the Lord and was put to shame?

Or whoever persevered in the fear of the Lord and was forsaken?

Or whoever called upon him and was overlooked?"[126]

When stressed, we are advised by Sirach not to be hasty in making decisions. Instead, we are encouraged to continue clinging to our higher power and to place our trust, hope, and confidence there. And then comes the promise of "everlasting joy." So here, in ancient wisdom, we have a continuum for relieving so much of the stress in our life and recapturing its joy: *Joy —> stress —> thinking through decisions —> clinging to God —> everlasting joy!*

Having considered joy, stress, and contemplation in our previous chapters, and armed with the wisdom of Sirach, we are ready to develop concrete ways to understand the nuances of our stress, to manage our way out of harmful stress, and to prepare ourselves to enter the presence of God. The managing of the stress aims at reducing it to a tolerable or creative level — but to stop there is not really to have experienced the joy within ourselves that is transformational and long lasting. I have been holding that it takes both — the stress management *and* the contemplative presence — for long lasting results.

We do not begin this chapter on managing stress without the prior exposure of some major contributions in this regard.[127] Over many of the psychological works on stress reduction, I have found Laurel Mellin, who is the Director of the National Research Coordinating Center for Emotional Brain Training at University of California at San Francisco's Center for Health and

---

[126] Sirach 2:2-3, 6, 8-9, 10, (Revised Standard Version).
[127] See Bibliography for Major Works on Stress Reduction, 189.

Community, to be the most applicable to my retreat work, where psychology and spirituality are combined. It is also the impressive melding of these two disciplines that were practiced in my years as a Spiritual Integrator at St. Luke Institute in Silver Spring, Maryland. However, while Mellin speaks of five states in which the brain can be, I have found it helpful in my work to reduce the five to three, namely States 1, 3, and 5. This is not to deny that her States 2 or 4 are not noteworthy. I simply believe three levels can serve well the task of "managing" what we are attempting to accomplish. Her three states are as follows:

> **State 1:** You're in the flow and your whole brain is in balance

> **State 3:** You are a little stressed and emotions are ramping up, particularly negative ones

> **State 5:** You are stressed out and over the top[128]

From here on, I will refer to these three states as No Stress, Medium Stress, and High Stress, the prior of which I would call, "Poised for Joy," because along with contemplative presence, both working together would complete the "reclaiming of joy" from which the title of this work is derived.

As a verb that takes an object, the verb manage means "to handle or direct with a degree of skill."[129] In this sense, we can manage our stress. As it is with managing anything like a project at work, a household task, or something regarding my personal life, before any managing can take place, I first have to understand my mental and emotional state, the task at hand, the resources I have, and very importantly, the steps it will take for me to get to the goal. There are deeper, more lasting ways of managing your stress that, when developed into a paradigm, can offer you a way inward to the joy that lies within you. It is not a joy you create, but one that was initially there at birth and continues to be present, although not experienced. The equation might look something like this: *Original joy —> life's stresses —> managing stress —> contemplative prayer —> recapture joy within.* Figure 7 Recapturing the Joy Within illustrates how the experience of extreme stress can find us at the base of a pyramid and how, through first, the managing of stress, we can ascend to a lessening level of stress and a greater readiness to God's presence within us. The working or grace is accessed through contemplative prayer, which literally takes us to the heights of prayer and union with God, represented by the pinnacle of the pyramid.

[128] Laurel Mellin, *Wired for Joy: A Revolutionary Method for Creating Happiness from Within,* (New York: Hays House, 2010), 105–107.
[129] Merriam Webster Dictionary, s.v. "manage," accessed March, 5, 2017, http://wwwmerriam-webster.com.

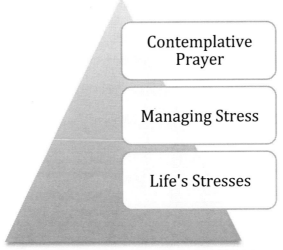

Figure 7 Recapturing the Joy Within

It is my intention that readers will, after reading this book, come away with a handy guide for understanding the particular stresses in their lives and practical ways to contact a deeper inner experience of joy.

SUMMARY OF HANDY GUIDES

What might such a guide look like and how might it be used? To achieve this goal, I have created several appendices, which can be copied and used as handy references. In them, the reader is provided with both theory and practices developed from practical application in past retreats that I have led.

Appendix A: Concerning Stress

Appendix B: How to Deal with Stress: 33 Tips That Work

Appendix C: 25 Classical Musical Works on Joy

Appendix D: 25 Poems on Joy

Appendix E: 10 Paintings on Joy

Appendix F: Concerning Contemplation

Appendix G: 5 Breathing Exercises to Lower Your
    Stress Levels

Appendix H: The State of Being Awake

Appendix I: 45 Fruits and Flowers of the Presence Practice

Appendix J: Concerning Planning

Appendix K: The Ignatian Examen as a Stress Reliever

Appendix L: Invitation to Join an Online Contemplative
    Prayer Group

These resources will serve the reader with both the theoretical and practical applications that were addressed directly or obliquely in the body of the book. It is hoped they would constitute a schematic outline of the steps for moving from stress to joy and the ability to both experience joy and maintain it for longer periods of time. It is, after all, what God wants for us!

STRESS AND STRESSORS; POSITIVE & NEGATIVE STRESS: WHAT'S THE DIFFERENCE?

Stress is our physiological or emotional response to a specific stimulus. I find it helpful to distinguish it from a "stressor," which is the actual thing creating the occasion for stress. Note that a stressor for one person may not be a stressor for another. Second, stress, as we have been saying all along, may be positive or negative based on its intensity. A moderate stress is motivating, whereas a great stress is not, and it will have harmful effects on the body. In all cases, stress responses are ways that help the body prepare for challenging situations. Let us take the example of having to postpone a large dinner party you were planning or for writing an article for a magazine. The dinner party or the article, when you first conceive it, is not in itself the stimulus for eventually getting the job done. However, the date or deadline, how challenging the task, and what must be done to prepare for it, will all have an impact on the level of stress you will experience. As the deadline draws near, and the degree that individual sub-tasks are or are not completed, will all determine how stressed you are feeling. Stress in such cases is seen as, "The mismatch between the perceived obstacle and the perceived resources for coping with the 'demands' of the obstacle."[130] Think of negative stresses on a scale of 1–5, with 5 being the greatest. On such a scale, a stress of 5 would be considered as beyond your control, and your mental, physiological, and emotional life is being strongly impacted negatively. At Level 3 (mild stress), we might experience the positive effects of stress, such as creativity or more efficient use of time and resources, both of which might result in a greater sense of self and improved self-esteem. The added benefit of moderate stress is that it helps us deal with slightly higher levels of stress that present themselves in the future in a positive way.

---

[130] "What is Stress," Explorable, accessed March 5, 2017, https://explorable.com/what-is-stress.

LEVELS OF STRESS AND INITIAL WAYS TO MANAGE THEM

Let us now turn to the author that has played a large part in my applying stress management to spiritual experience. She is the aforementioned Laurel Mellin. She holds that everyone's brain is in one of five states every moment of every day. These states are determined by the amount of cortisol that is dousing your prefrontal cortex,[131] which is the executive functioning section of your brain, causing your thinking to become extreme, chaotic, and rigid. In contrast to this dousing of cortisol, is the brain chemical called dopamine, which, rather than chaos, causes the prefrontal cortex to feel pleasure, fulfillment, and satisfaction. Her five states of the brain — three of which were mentioned earlier — relate to the amounts of cortisol or dopamine washing over the prefrontal cortex. The complete list of five is as follows:[132]

> **State 1:** You're in the flow and your whole brain is in balance
> **State 2:** You're slightly more stressed, but you feel balanced and generally good
> **State 3:** You're a little stressed and emotions are ramping up, particularly negative ones
> **State 4:** Definitely stressed and you're either ramping up emotions or shutting them down, depending on how your brain tends to process
> **State 5:** You're stressed out and over the top

MONDAY, WEDNESDAY, AND FRIDAY'S CHILD

To make things concrete, let us take the example of the parent of a Kindergartener. It is her first day of school. Off your little one goes, full of enthusiasm and joy over her new adventure with a ride on the big yellow bus. The day passes, and she comes home brimming with delight. She loves her new teacher and many of the friends from pre-school that she sees again.

---

[131] Some of the functions of the prefrontal cortex include: Coordinating and adjusting complex behavior, Impulse control and control and organization of emotional reactions, Focusing and organizing attention, Complex planning, and Considering and prioritizing competing and simultaneous information. The ability to ignore external distractions is partially influenced by the prefrontal cortex. It is generally agreed among neurologists that the prefrontal cortex does not fully develop until the age of 25. Is it any wonder that parents will often respond to a teen's strange behavior with the question, *"What were you thinking!"* The fact is, they were not thinking, nor did they have the full capacity to do so.

[132] Mellin, Op. cit., 105-107.

And look! She has done a finger painting, "Just for mommy." How does a parent respond? "Oh, honey, it's beautiful. Look at all the colors and shapes and action. Wow! Tell me about it?" As the child expresses her emotions, her parent draws them out affirming and augmenting them as well. So she responds with, "Let's put it on the refrigerator for all to see. Wait till grandma sees your very first finger painting," and on it goes. You have just witnessed what I would call "Monday's Child" as a way of linking Stage 1 to the first day of the week for easy remembering.

The week moves on, and it is now Wednesday. You're awaiting her with great expectations for another great day at school. In she comes, exclaiming, "We have homework, just like the big kids, but I don't know how to do it." "Was there something you didn't understand, honey?" you inquire. No response. She removes her backpack and opens the fridge for a snack. You repeat your question, and she begins to sadden. "Yes, everybody in the class knows, but I don't, and I was afraid to ask because they would make fun of me," she responds. You begin by noting her negative feelings of being made fun of, the risk involved, and her having to live with not knowing how to do the assignment. Then you switch to a more positive approach. You recall things she did not know at other times and how she would ask you about them or go to a friend. You remind her how good finally understanding made her feel. You suggest that she might ask her teacher when she is alone, and she could have the same good feeling again. But for now, you would help her understand. The conversation continues over milk and chocolate chip cookies. The antidote for your child experiencing moderate stress was simply to reflect the negative feelings she was experiencing and then the positive ones, past or present. Doing so helped her balance out her emotions, returning her to a state of calm. Let us name one in moderate stress "Wednesday's Child."

The week has moved on, and it is Friday. The first week of Kindergarten completed. It is 3:25 pm and in stomps your daughter, crying and shouting uncontrollably between her sobs, "It's not fair! It's not fair!" She throws her backpack across the kitchen floor and begins pounding on the table. What is a parent to do? You run to her and hold her tightly in your arms and *ask*, "What's not fair, my darling?" "I was pushed on the bus and made fun of because of my name," she sobs. I never want to go to school again! "Stay with me, sweetheart," you assure her. "I'm here; all will be okay. I'm here." The tantrum softens; the sobbing continues. Notice here that a caring parent, in embracing the child, is also controlling any possible further damage that might result from the tantrum. The loving embrace also serves as protection and reassurance to her. Words encouraging her that all is well, all will be well, are helpful for her to hear and to hear that this, too, will pass. "Friday's Child" was filled to overflowing with stress, and the parent exercised damage control, protection, and the reassurance that it would pass.

What comes naturally to a loving and sensitive parent is also good psychology for stress management. We will now look at each of the three stages of emotion and, with the example of the parent and Monday, Wednesday, and Friday's Child, see how we might better assist the child within us who is in either one of those three states. What we have developed so far is summed up in Figure 8.[133]

EMOTION EXPERIENCED	MANAGING IT
In Joy	Enjoy, savor, and enlarge it
In Moderate Stress	Name negative and positive feelings
In Great Stress	Exercise damage control or protection and reassurance that it will pass

Figure 8 Managing Three Levels of Emotion

BRINGING THE IDEAS HOME

Lest we remain in the world of the theoretical, I would like to apply the three levels on the stress/joy scale to a recent experience of my own as a way of understanding common stresses and common ways to reduce them. These "ways" were my own un-reflected ways of dealing with them at the time they occurred. I would then like to segue to Mellin's Emotional Brain Training methods that, very appropriately, offer the same advice from a scientific perspective. This is all to say that, if you are able to relieve stresses in your own life, then you may already be using very effective methods and have arrived at them naturally or intuitively. If that is the case, I would then encourage you to both confirm that as well and also remain open to adding new methods to your own tool kit. Just a reminder, the equation for recapturing the joy already within you is to recognize stress, have tools to manage it, move to an inner place of grace, move out of that space renewed, and work to sustain the joy for longer periods of time. Having had the experience empowers you to meet tomorrow's stressors when they surface.

---

[133] Ibid., 135–156.

EXAMPLES OF HIGH
OR MODERATE STRESS

We saw in Figure 1 — and we repeat the figure here — that some stress is important for performance.

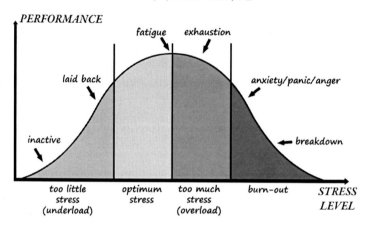

Figure 1 The Stress Curve

No stress characterizes performance as inactive or laid back. This is why, for example, we purchase a subscription to the theater, take out a membership in an athletic club, or make dinner engagements. If we left such things to the whim of the moment, we probably would never get around to doing them, and the fact remains, they are good, life-enhancing activities and satisfy the basic need we all have for affiliation and connection. There is within us, in the moment, a performance default that would have us just lie on our lily pad soaking up the sun. Yes, some stress is important for performance. The optimum amount of stress is that which gets us moving to be responsible and life-giving to others, and it peaks at the level of fatigue. When that point is reached, performance begins to decline into exhaustion. For our purposes, I will call high-level of stress as "too much stress" and moderate stress as "optimum stress." Normally, employing stress-reducing techniques in the latter case just short of fatigue is the best use of stress. More about this in a moment.

While Mellin lists five different levels on the stress-to-joy continuum, as mentioned above, I have found that in leading many retreats on the subject, the three levels of High Stress, Medium Stress, and No Stress are sufficient, while introducing step 1 as the bridge to lasting, transformational joy.[134] I believe that this is a contribution on my part to the symbiotic relationship of nature and grace, which will be the topic of Chapter 6.

For a "High Stress" example, permit me to recall a recent incident. I was to lead a parish retreat in Ocala, Florida. I got to Baltimore Washington International Airport a full two hours before the flight. This was my normal manner of doing things; I like to arrive at places early and keep busy in the car while I wait for the appointed time. In this case, I would use sitting at the gate as an opportunity to engage with my laptop and do some deskwork. After an hour, I gathered up my things and went to the men's room. Returning, I got my usual skinny latte, and I sat down at the gate again, very interested in returning to my opened documents. After a while, I felt myself getting drowsy and decided to just close my eyes a bit. The second hour passed as I dozed. Eventually, I was startled by an announcement regarding boarding. I looked up at the board, and my boarding time had passed and, much to my horror, the new boarding being called for was to Albany, NY! What! What had happened to my plane to Orlando? My heart began to thump, my face flushed, a sense of horror came over me. I hurriedly made my way to the gate desk and, very upset, had to wait my turn in line. Finally, the attendant! "What happened to the plane to Orlando?" I implored. "Orlando?" she replied. "The gate for that flight had been changed to gate 12 an hour ago." I realized I had slept through the gate change of my flight and the reassignment of the Albany flight to my gate.

How would I ever make it to Orlando in time, pick up my rental car, drive two hours to Ocala, check into the hotel, drive to the retreat site, and be ready to present by 4:00 pm? Never; I would never make it! Barely able to breathe, I asked the attendant, "When's the next plane to Orlando?" "Twelve fifteen," she replied, "I'd have to put you on stand-by; you'd be sixth in line." The breathing became more rapid; the heart rate began to increase again. "What's the likelihood of getting on?" I pleaded. "Not good, but I have a flight out at 4:00 with only two on standby." "Put me on the 12:15 as seventh in line," I said.

What was I going to do? I returned to my seat in the loading area feeling like I wanted to cry. Having arrived two hours early and now missing my plane…this just wasn't fair! "Get a grip; it isn't the end of the world. I'm still alive, am I not!" I said and began breathing deeply. As I did, alternatives began coming to mind: I could cancel the 4:00 session, add an extra session

[134] "2015 Stress in America," American Psychological Association, accessed December 5, 2016, http://www.apa.org/news/press/releases/stress/2015/snapshot.aspx.

on Sunday, or lengthen the Friday evening session. I stopped, got quiet, and decided to turn it all over to God. "Your will be done" rang in my ears. I remember asking, "Lord, help me to see the good in all this." After 10 or 15 minutes of resting in the silence, things began to open up. I wasn't quite ready to call Ocala to bring them in on what had happened. When I finally did, however, they assured me that they would hold me in prayer, and we worked out alternatives that also included regular texting updates from me the rest of the day and an alternative to the 4:00 pm session that did not include me, if that had to be.

What I would like to note at this point of my story, are the practices that came out of my way of doing things that addressed both the nature and grace that were operative in this extremely stressful situation. For nature, we had the breathing and self-talk like "It's not the end of the world," etc. For grace, we had the prayerful words, the silence, the turning it over, and the "Thy will be done" intention. Once I had settled down and regained a sense of calm and inner strength, I went back to my laptop and continued the work I had brought with me for the wait and the remote chance that I had to be on the 12:15 flight. What I felt most deeply was the reassurance that whether it was the 12:15 or the 4:00 or the 8:00 flight this evening, all would be well. Things certainly look different when emotions are tended to, and we allow God into our lives through contemplative presence.

Mellin explains well the State 5 stress that I experienced. She would understand well the things I did to bring me a sense of calm in what was initially experienced as a turbulent sea of emotions. When one is in Brain State 5, Mellin offers what she calls "The Damage Control Tool." It consists of repeating three specific phrases continuously until you actually feel a break in the spiral of emotions. The statements are: "Do not Judge," "Minimize Harm," and "Know It Will Pass."[135] She states, "All that the words do is remind you of the best strategies to use when the error of Brain State 5 emerges."[136] The first, "Do not Judge," reminds you in your state of being overwhelmed not to label anyone as bad, including yourself. Because you are out of control, it is an easy thing to do, but it gets you nowhere in terms of recovery. The second statement, "Minimize Harm," helps ease the spontaneous maladaptive behavior that you may well be considering, and the third, "Know It Will Pass," is an all-important reminder that this too shall pass; it is only a temporary state, horrendous though it may be. Mellin holds, and I have experienced this often myself, that the constant mental repetition of the statements does have an effect. It does quiet me down; it does reduce my stress level, and it returns me to a calmer state. It is as if the brain has turned down the faucet that is

[135] Mellin, Op. cit., 139.
[136] Ibid., 138.

splashing cortisol on my prefrontal cortex. No, I may not yet be experiencing a dopamine rush of joy, but I am somewhat less stressed. And to think, all it took was the repetition of a few phrases. The shift in emotion is indeed very real. Try it and you will become a believer in using this very simple, though effective tool.

Now let us consider a situation of a more moderate level of stress. For me, such situations are frequent. Misplacing my car keys, being unable to find my credit card, having a different expectation about vacation plans — these are things in my life that cause me moderate levels of stress. Mellin would call such a state, Brain State 3.[137] For this state, she also offers a tool to move you to a state of joy and calls it the "Emotional Housekeeping Tool." Here the person under stress is invited to fully express all his feelings about the issue causing the stress. This is clearly something that is not afforded the person in Brain State 5. It would have been dangerous to do so in those circumstances. She attests that most folks in State 3, and using the tool, can bring instant relief. She states:

> "This tool works so well because you are only a little stressed... You just need to offload a bit of stress. Stress is just excitations of neurons, and in Brain State 3, more neurons are activated. What is the best way to alleviate that stress? Express your emotions."[138]

This is how the Emotional Housecleaning Tool works. You begin by expressing any and all negative emotions you are feeling such as anger, sadness, fear, or guilt. Be complete; think of your response as a forced choice question on a survey. So regarding the loss of my car keys, I might have admitted to myself that, "I was angry for not paying more attention to where I put them; angry for not putting them in the only place I ever put them when they are not in my pocket; I feel sad that I'm an adult and that I am losing things like a child; I fear that I don't have a duplicate set; and I feel guilty that this isn't the first time this has happened."

You are then asked to shift to expressing positive emotions that involve gratitude, happiness, security, or pride. So I might say, "I feel grateful to have a friend to whom I can admit my foibles and happy that the keys have to be somewhere in the house and will eventually turn up; and secure that I can call the dealership to have another key issued; or relieved that my good reputation is not at stake." So, you get the idea. The result is that the person can move from a State of 3 to one of joy, a State of 1.

---

[137] Ibid., 140-141.
[138] Ibid., 140.

CRITICAL STRESS LEVELS

While many authors deal with stress reduction in a similar fashion, I was particularly taken by Lauren Mellin's approach. She is clear, concise, and graphic in the presentation of her theory. Although I have adhered to what she calls Level 1, 3, and 5 of her five stress levels, I have chosen not to highlight her Levels 2 and 4. As I have already mentioned, it is not so much that they are not important, but more that I am not sure that the nuancing they offer is critical. I have come to this position from my own experience of stress, and from a series of retreats I have conducted over three years on the subject. The other way I have digressed from Mellin is by adding the dimension of contemplative prayer to the equation as the way spiritual joy can be experienced and sustained. This latter was not a consideration of Mellin's, in that her approach was more psychological than spiritual.

MANAGING HIGH STRESS

In this stage, the individual is overwhelmed with emotion, so much so that they are unable to think critically, realize the impact of their emotion, or manage their behavior. They need internal and external assistance. If it is the case of "Friday's Child,"[139] and a caring individual is present, all the better. If it is the case of you as an adult, then the "adult" within you needs to take charge of your "inner child." As we saw previously, the child's mother embraces the ranting and raving youngster, an embracing that in effect minimizes the damage that the ranting could cause, while also offering her a non-judgmental response and an assurance that all will be well. This array of responses on the part of the mother Mellin calls the "Damage Control Tool." She offers it as a sort of narrative that the adult speaks to the inner child, though she does not use those exact words. For the reality of the words to break through, she suggests repeating the phrase 10-20 plus times, over and over, until it registers and breaks the circuit of anxiety. And, at one point, it decidedly will and, either joy will be experienced, or at least the individual will move out of stress Stage 5 to a lower level that can be handled by still another tool she will offer. Mellin presents Stage 5 and the Damage Control Tool as follows:[140]

---

[139] Ibid., 139.
[140] Ibid., 139.

IN BRAIN STATE 5, USE THE DAMAGE CONTROL TOOL TIME REQUIRED 2-5 MINUTES
1. Say, "Do not Judge" (myself or others)
2. Repeat (10-20 plus times)
3. Feel Surge of Joy

Figure 9 Damage Control Tool

It becomes very clear how the child's mother provides a portal for her to experience connection to a loving, caring world outside of her overwhelming anxiety and how this action begins the flow of dopamine. It also reduces the pain and suffering caused by the dousing of the prefrontal cortex with stress creating cortisol. While it may look a bit unbelievable, the repetition, when it "clicks," is amazing. Mellin refers to this "click" as "breaking the stress circuit and creating a joy circuit."[141] What works for mother and child, works for the adult and the inner child within me in such moments of extreme stress.

MANAGING MODERATE STRESS

I would like to discuss this Level 3 of stress as a very creative one, filled with the potential for motivation, direction, and anticipation of a job well done. We have already alluded to the fact that the strings of a violin can be stretched too tightly and snap — think Stage 5 — or so loose they cannot be played. However, there is in the process of tuning a point where the ear can sense the perfect balance of tension, where the note played is in perfect synchronization with the tuning instrument. Because it is all about balance — think of a see-saw of negatives and positives in balance, meeting on a perfect horizontal plane — we look critically while in this stage at all the positive and negative aspects of the emotions and see precisely what is out of balance. The individual in this state is free enough not to be hooked into a frenzied reaction of Stage 5, but better able to give a more measured response in Stage 3. Ah, the joy of a measured response!

---

[141] Ibid., 138.

What Mellin has done is to take the classic emotions, both negative and positive, and array them in a format of "I statements" that individuals at stress Level 3 can state about themselves. So, for the negative emotions of anger, sadness, fear, and guilt, one would assert: "I feel angry that...," "I feel sad that...," "I feel afraid that...," and "I feel guilty that..." The same is done for the other side of the emotional seesaw, namely, for grateful, happy, secure, and proud. Thus we have, "I feel grateful that...," "I feel happy that...," "I feel proud that..." As each feeling is expressed, stress should begin to decrease in intensity. If it does not, it may be that you have too much of it. Mellin suggests up to five statements for each feeling and, if it does not seem to fade, simply go on to the next feeling.[142] It is more than likely that responses to all the feelings will not be on the same topic that is arousing the feelings. Using this tool of balancing the see-saw, which Mellin calls "The Emotional Housecleaning Tool," you will eventually feel joy inasmuch as the stress has been reduced and the cortisol level decreased or gone, and the dopamine level is beginning to rise. Again, it should be noted that we are talking psychology not spirituality, which, I would hold, stabilizes and secures the possibility for an inner joy that serves to protect one against future assaults of stress. Figure 10 summarizes Mellin's Emotional Housecleaning Tool.

IN BRAIN STATE 3, USE THE EMOTIONAL HOUSECLEANING TOOL TIME REQUIRED 1 MINUTE
Express Negative Emotions *"I feel angry that..."* *"I feel sad that..."* *"I feel afraid that..."* *"I feel guilty that..."*
Express Positive Emotions *"I feel grateful that..."* *"I feel happy that..."* *"I feel secure that..."* *"I feel proud that..."*
Feel Surge of Joy

Figure 10 Emotional Housecleaning Tool

---

[142] Ibid., 142.

This balancing of positives and negatives helps one to reframe mentally what is perceived, and the consideration of both the positives and negatives does justice to allowing us to feel the entire field of our experience. Yes, there is light at the end of the tunnel! The so-called negative emotions are no longer seen as negative, but rather just "difficult" or "challenging," and more importantly, something that can be overcome. In this way, you are able to name the emotion, honor it, but not create a bias against the experience. What was perhaps a fate that you had to suffer through has become a challenge you can face, given the positive aspects that were also arising from the stressful situation.

MANAGING FOR JOY

As we have applied Levels 3 and 5, respectively, to Wednesday's and Friday's child,[143] we will now apply Level 1 to Monday's child and spell out in greater detail how this state is managed in order to experience it more fully. Recall the exuberance of the child's first day at Kindergarten and the excitement she felt regarding her very first finger painting. The parent made every effort to stay in the moment with the energy the youngster was experiencing. This was done by asking questions, sharing the joy and glee of the experience. Facial expressions, hugs, and an animated voice might have all accompanied the parent's sharing. An attempt was made to extend and augment the joy by speaking about sharing the finger painting with others in the home by posting it on the refrigerator, mentioning at the dinner table, or taking it to a sick or homebound relative to enjoy. This will certainly be one day this child will never forget. Analogously, the very same procedure would be followed with the adult and inner child of all your own State 1's. Stay in the moment, rest in it, relish, and savor it. If it was as simple a thing as washing and vacuuming out the car, return to it for an extending of the pleasure or joy. If it was cleaning out the closet, arranging the pantry, folding and storing the laundry, planting the garden, you name it, return and smile as you gaze again upon the completed word. Enjoy it, mentioning and sharing it with another, and return to it as often as you like for continuing joy. Figure 11 summarizes Mellin's Sanctuary Tool.

---

[143] See page 91.

IN BRAIN STATE 1, USE THE SANCTUARY TOOL TIME REQUIRED 20–30 SECONDS
1. Lovingly Observe Yourself Connect to the Safe Place Within
2. Feel Compassion for Yourself Feel Compassion for Yourself Feel Compassion for Yourself
3. Feel Surge of Joy

Figure 11 Mellin's Sanctuary Tool

CAN YOU HAVE "UNFELT" JOY?

Several years ago, I was at a Mass at which a cardinal was preaching on the subject of joy. I remember his speaking of the unfelt joy he had experienced recently. "Unfelt joy" I asked myself? Knowing him to be one that lives in his head rather than from his heart, I quickly discounted such a notion. Clearly, you cannot have unfelt joy if joy is an emotion. It appears to me that joy is not a thing or substance that one reaches out and takes hold of. Yet, it is something you can possess and experience. How do you reconcile the discrepancy? You might think of joy as a capacity, a womb-like situation wherein the individual can receive a new life, a new experience. In such a scenario, the "seed" that is needed for the joy-experience is to be stress-less and in the presence of God. Thus, it is the person's soul or spirit that is "cleared for conception," if you will, where the spark of life is ignited by God, and the joy is experienced!

BRINGING THE IDEAS HOME

Let us return to Monday, Wednesday, and Friday's child one last time. This image was used as illustrative of the tools that are readily available to you in any of the three states. They are as easy to apply, as it is to care for a youngster exhibiting behavior indicative of any of the states. The application comes naturally and is intuitive. Simply extend those same intuitive tools as the adult to your inner child, and you will have what is needed in the moment. Yes, it is possible to move from high stress to moderate stress, and then from moderate stress to joy in a matter of minutes without the use of medication, excessive snacking, or employing any other substance to dull the pain. Stress is indeed constructive, if you know how to manage it.

GETTING STRESS
TO WORK FOR YOU

Our culture today tends to support a lie about stress and tension, namely, that it is always bad and that happiness is the only goal before us. Happiness or joy is not something we can achieve and have last 24/7. That is because we are human and limited, and it is also because we are social beings in relationship with others, and there are bound to be different opinions about almost any subject. However, to be human is to adapt and grow, as is true of any living thing. To be in relationship with others is to experience life-giving affiliation. It would be like asking the violin to play without a well-proportioned tension in its strings. There is a real downside to living without a modicum of stress. It can make us a bit gullible and trusting, thinking all is well,

> "Research shows that when we're overly happy, our comfort with the status quo interferes with our ability to attend to detail as we 'let the good times roll.' Sometimes we need to be able to sacrifice short-term happiness to accomplish more meaningful long-term goals, but that can be harder to do if you make happiness a priority."[144]

Tolerating and working with moderate levels of anger, anxiety, and stress can prepare us for major stressful situations, and they can also serve as motivators to move on a project or meet a deadline. Is it not important to feel the discomfort or stress in walking down a dark street alone? Is it not good to express anger when someone is being bullied or taken advantage of? And what of the frustration and stress in not having been able to complete something by a deadline? Does it not open you up to a renewed sense of commitment? Moderate levels of stress are excellent red flags that something is not right in a situation and that we need to act. "Every emotion is useful – even the ones we think of as negative. Without them we would be living in a world devoid of fully functioning human beings."[145]

WHERE IS GOD IN ALL THIS?

It is as if we now stand on the threshold or watershed between stress reduction and experiencing spiritual joy. Before moving on to Chapter

---

[144] Todd Kashdan and Robert Biswas-Diener, "Join the grouchy club: Why negative emotions can be a force for good," *Mail Online*, last modified January 3, 2015, accessed March 15, 2017, http://www.dailymail.co.uk/home/you/article-2894291/Join-grouchy-club-negative-emotions-force-good.html.

[145] Ibid.

6 and a consideration of the Nature/Grace reality in the life of the believer, I wish to share a little piece of folklore I learned from my mother. Whenever we children were in a snit over things not going our way or our expectations being unfulfilled, her response usually included two parts: "It wasn't meant to be," and "Where is God in this?" Belief in those two statements came easy because of the faith we had in our mother, and they helped us sit a bit with the stress or heartbreak. More importantly, they gave us the space to look what God's plan for the upset might have been. While I was only a pre-teen when I first received this maternal wisdom, it was their repetition during my formative years that laid the foundation for years of applications, applications that continue to this day.

STRESS LEVELS 5 AND 3 AS PORTALS TO CONTEMPLATION AND RESULTING JOY

In reading the literature of psychologists, one might come to the conclusion that once stress is handled and lowered, that a state of nirvana ensues. I believe this to be true in part, but the whole truth is that the joy that bubbles up from within the individual has another source, and it is a spiritual one at that. At this time in our culture, an education beyond the head, one that also includes the heart, is needed. Mystics from all faith traditions testify to this in the way they deal with stress, their practice of some form of spiritual unity, and the expression of the presence in the quality of their choices and their living with others. It is the task of this book to link the three together as a way of reclaiming the capacity for primordial joy within us, a joy that gives us a lasting foundation for peace, purpose, and passion. Stress has a way of dampening our spirits and imprisoning our minds. How easy it is to forget who we are and why we are here. We have been created for joy and to live in joy. The extraordinary gift of joy, once experienced, is that we come to know that joy is enough; we have enough. Nothing more is needed.

What lies deep within the individual is a God-given natural state. It is a state that was masked and covered over with the accumulated stress of years. Stress reduction, be it movement from a Level 5 (high stress) to 3 (moderate stress), or a Level 3 to 1 (joy), becomes the springboard for a richer, more fulfilling, more stable experience of grace and transformation.

In his book, *Return to Joy,* Andrew Harvey writes, "What is needed for all of us is to find the way back to what all spiritual traditions know as the essence of reality — the simple joy of being that is the indispensable foundation for all meaningful living and all truly effective action."[146]

---

[146] Andrew Harvey and Carolyn Baker, *Return to Joy,* (Bloomington: iUniverse, 2016), xxiii.

MOVEMENT FORWARD
IN THE LITERATURE

At this point, it might serve us well to cite two contributions I hope this work may be making to the literature. In Chapter 3 on contemplation, I attempted to add to Keating's thoughts on Centering Prayer by using the breath more effectively, that is, by deep breathing till complete relaxation is achieved. This would make it easier to keep the mind from thinking and giving in to distractions. In addition, the sacred word could be one or two words, but no more than four syllables and synchronized to the breathing. This is contrary to Keating's thinking that the word is not a mantra and need not be repeated. A second movement forward came in condensing Mellin's five stages to three for easier application and the use of the Monday, Wednesday, and Friday's child, as an easy way to remember the steps and what appropriate applications might be.

MAINTAINING THE JOY WITHIN

Perhaps one of the most well-known and familiar faces of joy is Pope Francis. The joy radiates in his smile with anyone he meets. No one is a stranger; no one is excluded. It is not an accident that his stunning encyclical Laudato Si' has been called one of the most profound works on spiritual ecology and responsible stewardship of the earth. He has challenged world leaders and all people to care for the earth as our common home. It should also be noted that despite this exuberance of joy, he has received from cardinals, bishops, and the Roman Curia a great deal of pushback on many of his reforms to bring this face of joy and compassion to the Church-at-large. When asked how he handles his stress he remarks, "I don't let it bother me." Being able not to take it seriously, maintaining a rich prayer life, and moving from joy to compassionate and caring action are all part of how he serves his God and the world. In a homily he gave at World Youth Day in 2013 he said, "And here the first word that I wish to say to you: Joy! Do not be men and women of sadness: A Christian can never be sad! Never give way to discouragement! Ours is not a joy born of having many possessions, but of having encountered a Person: Jesus, in our midst."[147]

In these times, it is becoming clearer that we need not only to reduce our levels of stress dramatically, but we also need to have practical ways to return to "the joy of our youth," as we used to say in the old form of the Catholic Mass.[148] The joy of our youth is precisely the kind of joy that one can

---

[147] Pope Francis, "Homily of Pope Francis," accessed March 15, 2017, http://w2.vatican.va/
content/francesco/en/homilies/2013/documents/papa-francesco_20130324_palme.html.
[148] The following prayer was said at the foot of the altar: *"And I will go to the altar of God: to God who gives the joy of my youth."*

experience in contemplative prayer, as we have seen. And not only has the stress been addressed, but any remaining stress can be held in prayer and let go of as an offering. In the presence, the freeing of one's spirit to simply be, and be with and in God, can have a healing and transformative effect.

REALIZATION OF GOSPEL JOY

It is safe to say that we are all born with a capacity to experience joy. It is a natural state that is achieved with most infants, who have not yet been tainted or wounded, and attested to by their nonverbal wiggling and giggling over almost anything crossing their path. Their joy is expressed in their never-ending excitement for contact with anything that is new. All senses are drawn to almost any object, as the infant struggles to make itself one with whatever is before him. And the longing continues throughout life. The Germans call this longing Sehnsucht.[149] C.S. Lewis, in his partial autobiography entitled *Surprised by Joy,* describes his journey in becoming a Christian. *Surprised by Joy* is an allusion to the poem by William Wordsworth entitled, "Surprised By Joy — Impatient As The Wind," which relates to the incident of Wordsworth forgetting the death of his dear daughter. The poem reads:

Surprised by joy — impatient as the Wind

I turned to share the transport — Oh! with whom

But Thee, deep buried in the silent tomb,

That spot which no vicissitude can find?

Love, faithful love, recalled thee to my mind —

But how could I forget thee? Through what power,

Even for the least division of an hour,

Have I been so beguiled as to be blind

To my most grievous loss? — That thought's return

Was the worst pang that sorrow ever bore,

Save one, one only, when I stood forlorn,

Knowing my heart's best treasure was no more;

That neither present time, nor years unborn

Could to my sight that heavenly face restore.[150]

---

[149] *Sehnsucht* is a German noun translated as "longing," "pining," "yearning," or "craving," or in a wider sense a type of "intensely missing." *Sehnsucht* is difficult to translate adequately and describes a deep emotional state.

[150] William Wordsworth, "Surprised by Joy," Poetry Foundation, accessed March 16, 2017, https://www.poetryfoundation.org/poems-and-poets/poems/detail/50285.

Lewis writes not to provide a chronicle of his life, but more to share what was for him the extraordinary discovery of joy. So lofty, yet so close, he was not able ever to put the experience into words. These "stabs of joy," as he referred to them, continued throughout his life in his journey from atheism to theism and finally to Christianity. I site an infant and then C.S. Lewis because the journey of joy is universal and gets specified in the adult. I believe it reaches its zenith in Christian contemplation. Lewis, in the end, does experience the true nature and purpose of joy and the place it is to have in his own life. As the book closes, Lewis realizes that joy can be a signpost on a tree in the woods where someone is lost. While it is not yet contained in its fullness, you share in some degree the joy of knowing you're on the way. And yet, because it is joy, it is at the same time enough and inexplicable!

LIVING THE DAY IN JOY

How is one to live in joy as a steady daily experience? At this point in our consideration of moving from stress to joy, I would say it takes noticing your level of stress, using tools appropriate to the level, and then moving into contemplative prayer. Chapter 6 will take up the relationship of the physiological and spiritual, that is, nature and grace. Finally, Chapter 7 will consider how being less stressed and in touch with the divine opens you up to being there for others.

ARRIVING AT THE JOY WITHIN

Joseph Campbell, the famous American Mythologist, lectured and wrote on comparative religious experiences. An often-quoted passage of his speaks of this joy, which we are desirous of reclaiming as our own. He writes:

"People say that what we're all seeking is a meaning for life. I don't think that's what we're really seeking. I think that what we're seeking is an experience of being alive, so that our life experiences on the purely physical plane will have resonances with our own innermost being and reality, so that we actually feel the rapture of being alive."[151]

With that we move on to the nature/grace bridge to the experience of "rapture."

---

[151] Joseph Campbell, *The Power of Myth,* (New York: Anchor Publishing, 1991), 84.

Reflection Questions for Chapter 5: Stress Relieving Techniques

- *What intrigues you most about stressors and how to manage them?*

- *List three times you have been at Stress Level of 5 and three times you have been at Stress Level of 3.*

- *How have the tools proper to each of the three levels (Level 5: Damage Control Tool, Level 3: Emotional Housecleaning Tool, Level 1: Sanctuary Tool) been helpful to you?*

- *When do you find some stress helpful to you?*

Chapter 6:
The Nature/Grace Reality
In the Life of the Believer

INTRODUCTION

We have come a long way — from an initial understanding of Christian joy to seeing how stress can block or conceal that joy. Contemplation, perhaps the deepest and most intimate of all prayer forms, was introduced in Chapter 4, and then we moved on to considering stress-relieving techniques as a way to get more easily into the experience of that joy already within an individual. This brings us to our present chapter and the consideration of how nature and grace are at work, not just in anyone, but also more specifically in the life of one who believes in God's immanent presence.

You may remember that we discussed the interplay of Nature and Grace in Chapter 1. What we need to add now is the impact of Nature and Grace *in the Life of the Believer.* That is to say that, in addition to a deeper understanding anyone could gain from consideration of the subject, what a Christian believer can add is an experience of those intellectual insights that are grounded in one's very belief in a Triune God. It is resting in this experience that calls forth joy of extraordinary proportions.

The connection between experience of a Triune God in contemplative prayer and the joy that lies within was made very clear to me by Richard of St. Victor, a Medieval Scottish philosopher and theologian (d. 1173). He states:

> "For God to be good, God can be one. For God to be loving, God has to be two. Because love is always a relationship. But for God to share excellent joy and delight, God has to be three, because supreme happiness is when two persons share their common delight in a third something — together."[152]

This joy within them is borne of a Triune God. Grace is part and parcel of the very nature of our being and moves all that exists forward toward growth and flourishing. It is our destiny to become all we are capable of being. It is quite literally the law of nature.[153] Our union with the Trinity as One, thus draws us inexorably into the joy of the Godhead itself. In our final chapter, we shall use the words of Richard of St. Victor to see the connection between Trinity, contemplative prayer, and contemplative action.

---

[152] Richard of St. Victor, *Richard of St. Victor: The Twelve Patriarchs, The Mystical Ark, Book Three of the Trinity,* (Classics of Western Spirituality), (Mahwah: Paulist Press, 1979), 387–389.
[153] Richard Rohr with Mike Morrell, *The Divine Dance: The Trinity and Your Transformation,* (New Kensington: Whitaker House, 2016), 158.

REMOVING THE VEIL

Paul speaks to the Christians at Corinth about this experience of Trinity,

> "When I was a child, I spoke like a child, I thought like a child, I reasoned like a child; when I became an adult, I put an end to childish ways. For now, we see in a mirror, dimly, but then we will see face to face. Now I know only in part; then I will know fully, even as I have been fully known. And now faith, hope, and love abide, these three; and the greatest of these is love.[154]

The believer comes to contemplative prayer with the knowledge and experience of having encountered God before. The silence of his prayer will be a union of hearts, a resting in the dynamic presence of the Trinity, as love of the three Persons overflows into the experience of the person in prayer. Removing the veil or "seeing more clearly in a mirror," as other translations would have it, deepens the experience of joy. C.S. Lewis has defined joy as feeling, "An intense overwhelming desire for an indefinable numinous something" that was just beyond his grasp. It was intimation to some higher reality. He continues, "If you try to hold on to the feeling of joy as an end in itself, it would vanish."[155] No, it is not about grasping for or even creating joy. It is about disposing oneself to God and surrendering to Trinitarian engagement that overflows into the experience of the believer. The experience, as it is taking place, is not articulated intellectually as understanding. It is experienced, and, only *after* it has ended and one has reflected on what happened, can it be described. After all, to describe it as it is taking place is to be engaged in thought, which would clearly take you out of the unitive experience, where there is no separation of thinker and object thought.

PORTALS OF JOY

Apart from stress and stress relievers, apart from contemplative practice, there are myriads of portals or openings that can access our joy directly. Anything of beauty, created by an artist or by the divine creator as in nature, can be such a portal. What comes to mind immediately are poems, paintings, and musical compositions. The following, which are my own top two

---

[154] 1 Corinthians 13:11-13, (New Revised Standard Version).
[155] Professor Louis Marko, *The Life and Writings of C. S. Lewis (The Great Courses)*, CD, (The Teaching Company, 2000).

contemplative favorites in the areas of poetry, music, and art, are offered, as it were, as analogous to *jolts* of breathing pure oxygen that might create a sense of euphoria when inhaled deeply. Appendices C, D, and E offer lengthier lists in all three categories for you, the reader.

From Poetry

"The Rose" by Theodore Roethke

> Near this rose, in this grove of sun-parched, wind-warped madronas,
>
> Among the half-dead trees, I came upon the true ease of myself,
>
> As if another man appeared out of the depths of my being,
>
> And I stood outside myself
>
> Beyond becoming and perishing,
>
> A something wholly other,
>
> As if I swayed out on the wildest wave alive,
>
> And yet was still.
>
> And I rejoiced in being what I was.[156]

"The Golden Echo" by Gerard Manley Hopkins

> Deliver it, early now, long before death,
>
> Give beauty back, beauty, beauty, beauty, back to God, beauty's
>
> Self and beauty's giver.[157]
>
> And in another place:
>
> This, all this beauty blooming,
>
> This, all this freshness fuming,
>
> Give God while worth consuming.[158]

---

[156] Theodore Roethke, "The Rose," *The Collected Poems of Theodore Roethke*, (New York: Anchor Books, 1974).

[157] Gerard Manley Hopkins, "The Golden Echo," Bartleby.com, accessed April 5, 2017, http://www.bartleby.com/122/36.html.

[158] Gerard Manley Hopkins, "Morning Midday and Evening Sacrifice," accessed April 5, 2017, http://www.famouspoetsandpoems.com/poets/gerard_manley_hopkins/poems/13995.

From Music

"The Lark Ascending" by Vaughan Williams

Written in 1914, its premiere had to be put on hold because of the outbreak of WWI. It was not performed until 1921. The soaring violin melody ascends so high that it is barely audible. To it, add the shimmering strings and the poignantly beautiful accompaniment, and what is called forth is the rolling English countryside. In the orchestral section, the lark returns, melodically entwining itself around the orchestra, but then breaking free and rising to still loftier heights. I experience it as the self, breaking free of the body in pure consciousness and uniting with the divine.[159]

"Méditation" from the opera *Thaïs* by Jules Massenet

The piece is written for solo violin and orchestra as part of the opera by the same name. It premiered in Paris on March 16, 1894. The "Méditation" is an instrumental entr'acte performed between the scenes of Act II in the opera Thaïs. In the first scene of Act II, Athanaël, a Cenobite monk, confronts Thaïs, a beautiful and hedonistic courtesan and devotée of Venus, and attempts to persuade her to leave her life of luxury and pleasure and find salvation through God. It is during a time of reflection following the encounter that the "Méditation" is played by the orchestra. In the second scene of Act II following the "Méditation," Thaïs tells Athanaël that she will follow him to the desert.

---

[159] Richard Brittain, "Vaughan Williams ~ The Lark Ascending," YouTube, accessed April 6, 2017, https://www.youtube.com/watch?v=ZR2JlDnT2l8.

From Art

The Promenade by Marc Chagall

This is one of the pictures that Chagall painted while on a home visit to Belarus from Paris. When he came in 1914, war broke out, and he could not return. In 1917, he was living back in Vitebsk. It was also the year he became engaged to Bella. Flying in the air celebrates the joy and ecstasy of their love. Bella is lifted into the air; they have left earth altogether. In *The Promenade,* she is clearly flying like a kite. He stands on the ground, holding her hand as she is pulled up into the air and tugged powerfully away from him by the wind. Her torso acts as the kite-sail, her legs playing freely in the air like a kite-tail dancing in the breeze.[160]

The Joy of Life by Henri Matisse

In 1906, Henri Matisse finished what is often considered his greatest Fauve painting, the *Bonheur de Vivre*, or the *Joy of Life*. It is a large-scale painting depicting an Arcadian landscape filled with brilliantly colored forest, meadow, sea, and sky and populated by nude figures both at rest and in motion. As with the earlier Fauve canvases ("Fauve" is a style of painting with vivid expressionistic and non-naturalistic use of color that flourished in Paris), color is responsive only to emotional expression and the formal needs of the canvas, not the realities of nature. The references are many, but in form and date, *Bonheur de Vivre* is closest to Cézanne's last great image of bathers.[161]

---

[160] "Marc Chagall," Yahoo Answers, accessed April 7, 2017, https://answers.yahoo.com/question/index?qid=20100203082601AACbpVi.

[161] Henri Matisse, "The Joy of Life," Wikiart, accessed April 17, 2017, https://www.wikiart.org/en/henri-matisse/the-joy-of-life-1906.

BEING RECEPTIVE AND OPEN
AND FREE OF STRESS

What you know in your head will never satisfy the deepest longings of your heart, nor will dogma ever satisfy for the direct experience of the divine that comes through contemplative presence and the joy that flows from that. We have seen how poetry, music, and art take you to the experience of joy directly without much "headwork" needed. And what each art form will call forth is prior images and former direct experiences. Why else would museums, concert halls, and poetry readings continue to be so popular? Art, broadly understood, and contemplative prayer in particular, are direct participations in the life of God. What flows is the grace, the energy that moves and sustains the universe. And the deep joy that is felt, not only draws us into communion with God, but with all other explications of that divine presence in created matter as well. "It is thus that we become by grace what God is by nature."[162] The mystics are very clear that once you attempt to know someone solely with your mind, you necessarily create an object/subject relationship and thus lose the very unity you are seeking. To really "know" someone is to enter into a living, thriving back-and-forth, give-and-take interaction. It has often been called a "mutual mirroring" that goes, "subject to subject, center to center, love to love."[163]

THE KINGDOM OF HEAVEN
AS THIS INNER EXPERIENCE

While many, if not most Christians, think of the Kingdom of Heaven as being a place one goes after death, the Evangelist Matthew offers his own corrective in contradicting that notion when he says, "The Kingdom of Heaven is within you." "Within you" is *not* "out there" or "later" when you die. If it is within and now, the experience must be attainable. So rather than dying into it, one awakens into it. Nor is the Kingdom a utopia of some sort. Heaven knows — pun intended — many attempts at creating a utopia have been tried, each promising the world, and each failing miserably. To that must be added the fact that Jesus also rejected any such state of the world. Recall when his followers wanted to make him king, he was strong and unequivocal. "My kingdom is not of this world." (John 18:36) When his followers wanted to proclaim him the Messiah, the divinely-anointed King of

---

[162] Catherine Mowry LaCugna, *God For Us: The Trinity and Christian Life,* (New York: HarperSanFrancisco, 1991), 1.

[163] Richard Rohr, "Knowing through Loving," Richard Rohr's Daily Mediation, February 16, 2017, accessed April 17, 2017, https://cac.org/knowing-through-loving-2017-02-26/.

Israel who would inaugurate the reign of God's justice upon the earth, Jesus shrank from all of it saying strongly and unequivocally, "My kingdom is not of this world" (John 18:36).

Where is it, then, one might ask? Jim Marion insightfully suggests that the Kingdom of Heaven is a metaphor for a *state of consciousness.* That is, it is not so much a place you go, but a place from which you *come.*[164] It is a more radical way of looking at the world, a transformed awareness, and it makes the experience of the world very different.[165] The awareness and resulting joy of contemplative prayer admit no separation between God and us, nor any separation between or among human beings.

SHEDDING THE FINAL OBSTACLE OF JOY: THE EGO

Somehow it does not make sense to say you have to get out of the way in order to achieve your goal. Such a dictum may be true of a project or course of action you need to take, since you are the source of the action and all is dependent on your participation. However, in the realm of relationships with others or with God, the dictum is perhaps less true. You do indeed need to get out of the way. As we will see next, consciousness and the real self are not those things that distinguish me from others, that is, the things that make us unique or different. This sense of the self is more of a mirage or an illusion. My real self is more the center that I share with others. Recall the realms of poetry, music, and art that lift me to union and comm-union. Prayer and joy call us to that center beyond ego, so the "who I am" is a "we." We do have the capacity to shift our noticing and our awareness to an entirely different base of perception, to live out of a different worldview, if you will. All we need to do is focus elsewhere and, as I said, "get out of the way."

GOING DEEPER: THE BRAIN'S JOY CENTER

Antonio Damasio, a neuroscience researcher, has shown how the brain creates consciousness. He begins by asking what consciousness is, that is, what is it we lose when we fall into dreamless sleep or go under anesthesia, and, upon waking, we regain. Knowing how our minds operate will help us better understand consciousness and from that, grasp a clearer understanding of contemplation and the joy that comes of it.

---

[164] Jim Marion, *Putting on the Mind of Christ: The Inner Work of Christian Spirituality,* (Charlottesville: Hampton Roads Publishing Company, 2000).
[165] Ibid.

Using its neurons, the mind creates a visual or auditory grid by which it can experience the external world. The images on these grids can then be stored and recalled from memory, recreating the original images and recreating the original experience. In his TED Talk of March 2011,[166] Damasio then considers how we develop a sense of self, one that is quite stable and does not vary from one day to the next. This sense of self begins with what we have within us that is stable. This stable center is our physical body. And while the parts of our bodies are different and grow at varying rates, the sense of who we are does not. The self affords us a sense of unity and continuity over time that is rooted in our physicality.

Dr. Damasio states, "There is a very tight coupling between the regulation of our body within the brain and the body itself, unlike any other coupling."[167] This bond is maintained permanently. Between the cerebral cortex, located just behind the forehead, and the spinal cord that begins in the upper neck or the base of the skull, is the all-important brain stem. It is the brain stem that encases the many life-regulating structures of the entire body. Injure the *upper* part of the brain stem, and you will exist in a comatose or vegetative state. Your mind and consciousness are gone. There is no longer a sense of self. However, lose the function of the *lower* part of the brain stem, and you will be completely paralyzed, but your consciousness will be maintained. Imprisoned within their own bodies, such persons are able to think and know. He continues,

> "It is out of this and out of this tight coupling between the brain stem and the body that I believe — and I could be wrong, but I don't think I am — that you generate this mapping of the body that provides the grounding for the self and that comes in the form of feelings…"[168]

So why is this of interest to us when considering contemplation and the resulting experience of joy? In Chapter 3, when we considered contemplation, you will recall that we used the tools of deep breathing and a word or two as a mantra. The repetitive breathing, *as a function of the body,* and the repetition of the mantra, *as a function of the cerebral cortex,* both allowed us entry into the brain stem, the former from below the brain stem, and the latter from above it. Both slipping away as we floated into awareness, we were able to find ourselves at the very seat of our consciousness, our sense of self, without thought and without intentional bodily functioning. Here, then, we were experiencing, though not in our thoughts or emotions,

---

[166] Antonio Damasio, "The Quest to Understand Consciousness," TED Talk, March 2011, accessed April 18, 2017, https://www.ted.com/talks/antonio_damasio_the_quest_to_understand_consciousness.

[167] Ibid., segment at 11:07.

[168] Ibid., segment at 13:27.

our deepest sense of self, our *being* with no *doing* on our part. In this inner sanctum, we were one with the energy that transcends all being and all beings — the very heart of God. The exchange of consciousness that is taking place at this level is the very nature of divine life. And because all things that exist share in this giving and receiving, they share in the joy of consequent union. Michael Brown writes in *The Presence Process,* "Giving-as-receiving is the energetic frequency upon which our universe is aligned. All other approaches to energy exchange immediately cause dissonance and disharmony in our life experience."[169] Obviously, it becomes imperative to look at the latest developments in neuroscience, as we have just done, to help us understand the power and experience of contemplation.

THE CHRIST BEYOND JESUS

There is, for the Christian believer, a rich relationship that grounds our own humanity to the world of spirit. It helps both to understand and experience the fruit of contemplative prayer and appreciate its flowering into compassionate care of creation, be it expressed as human, vegetative, or mineral in nature. The relationship is the incarnate nature of Jesus Christ. Many Christians have erroneously come to understand that "Christ" is in some way the last name of Jesus. That connotation takes us nowhere. However, when we think of Jesus as the incarnate son of God, one like us in all things save sin, we have a compassionate human being with whom to relate, one who knows the trials and tribulations, the joys and ecstasies of our daily living. But there is more! Because Jesus is also "The Christ," the long awaited Messiah, he is also cosmic in nature. In this realm of the cosmic, he is also the eternal word of the creator God. Here, he has existed from all time and for all time. Here, he is the Word that brought calm out of the chaos in the Genesis account of creation. Here, he is the substance and foundation of all that is and will be. As cosmic, Christ is beyond the limitations of humans' ability or inability to believe. To deny this grounding in the Cosmic Christ would be as foolhardy as denying that we need air to breathe or that plants need the sun to create photosynthesis. Jesus lived his humanity from the ground up. He woke up each morning and placed his feet on the ground, as do we all. In contemplative prayer, we too live from the ground up in much the same way. The thoughts and feelings associated with the day pass before us, and they either disturb, excite, concern, or relieve us. But our feet are on the ground, so wc do not fly off the handle, or get caught in the flywheel of our activities, as it were. It is specifically in Jesus, then, that we have begun our day. As we dispose ourselves to enter contemplation, we move from the Jesus

---

[169] Michael Brown, *The Presence Process,* (Vancouver: Namaste Publishing, 2005), 246.

of Nazareth, "one like us in all things," to the Cosmic Christ, "one who reigns over all creation," regardless of where individuals are in their personal belief or disbelief. James Finley puts it well, when he says,

> "There are not two minds of Christ, one human and the other divine. Rather, the mind of Christ is *the realized oneness of the divine* [emphasis mine] and all that we are as human beings. Who we are in Christ is in no way reducible to our everyday, ordinary self. Nor is who we are in Christ in any way dualistically other than our ordinary self."[170]

With contemplative practice, spiritual awakening continues to deepen, and the rhythm of Jesus/Christ, the human/the divine, my life/my prayer, becomes more habitual, until it comes full circle, as Finley describes it, and "We get up in the morning and touch our feet to the floor. And we know that this ordinary experience of this utterly ordinary event is the mystery of oneness with God manifesting itself in and as this very ordinariness."[171]

LIVING OUT OF THE COSMIC CHRIST

A reality that has come home to me helps me live out this Jesus of Nazareth/Cosmic Christ reality in my daily life, and I would like to share it with you. There is within me a wounded child. He is the youngster who was always chosen last when choosing sides for baseball because he was left-handed and was not able to play well. He is the child who had thoughts and images, dreams, and fantasies he didn't dare share with an adult, nor could he find another child with whom to share them. And so this inner life of rejection loomed large as he matured. This child still exists. It is my daily reminder that I am grounded in my humanity, and my feet are on the ground — the same ground on which I stood as a child. However, things have changed since those early days. I am able to also live out of a cosmic sense of Christ. Moving into contemplative prayer, I am able to go from "feet on the ground" to "heart in the air," be refreshed and return to the ground renewed. Then I am able to tend, heal, and caress, the child within me, and with the passage of each month and year the tending necessity is diminished until there is no need for apologies, suppression, or deep dark secrets. Powerlessness and shame are gone. I have moved from the "Jesus of Nazareth" to the "Cosmic Christ" and back to the "Jesus of Nazareth," renewed. This same compassionate love I can offer the

---

[170] Richard Rohr, "Being Human," Richard Rohr's Daily Meditation, February 21, 2017, accessed April 20, 2017, https://cac.org/being-human-2017-02-21/.
Adapted from James Finley, *Christian Meditation: Experiencing the Presence of God*, (New York: HarperSanFrancisco, 2004), 116, 121, 191-192.
[171] Ibid.

child in me becomes available to any and all who are hurting — a reality that now becomes more obvious from and through my own experience of woundedness and healing. Finley sums this up beautifully in a meditation entitled, "Dreaming Compassion."

> "To be transformed in compassionate love does not mean that you do not have to continue struggling and working through your shortcomings and difficulties. It means learning to join God who loves you through and through in the midst of all your shortcomings. As you continue to be transformed in this way, you come to realize that right here, right now, just the way you are, you are one with love that loves you and takes you to itself just the way you are."[172]

LIVING DAILY IN STATES OF JOY

If you are seeking, seek us with joy

For we live in the kingdom of joy.

Do not give your heart to anything else

But to the love of those who are clear joy.

Do not stray into the neighborhood of despair,

For there are hopes: they are real, they exist —

Do not go in the direction of darkness —

I tell you: suns exist

– Rumi

I would take Rumi at his word. Look carefully at what gives you joy and what clearly does not; then follow where the joy leads. In this same vein, Joseph Campbell used the expression, "Follow your bliss."[173] Trust your instincts in this regard. When and if the darkness of despair looms on the horizon, turn and walk away, be it the atmosphere, relationship, or mood you are in. Suns do exist! Spend time in them. In an act of self-disclosure, I have listed the top 10 things I spend time doing, many on most days, all at least every week that contribute to "following my bliss."

1.   The joy of solitude: The quiet hours before anyone arises at home or in the monastery, and I am able to draw a first steaming cup of coffee and simply sit.

---

[172] Ibid., 283–286.

[173] Joseph Campbell, *The Power of Myth*, (New York: Anchor Books, 1991), 120, 149.

2.   The joy of resting in nature: Walking slowly on the monastery grounds or up and down our very long and winding driveway without a destination in mind and encountering a squirrel looking at me and expecting acorns.

3.   The joy of being with and resting in friends (free of "catching up" and idle chatter): Sitting quietly with Michael, David, and John before a fire enjoying a glass of wine with long pauses between our shifting topics of spirituality, philosophy, or a piece of music or poetry.

4.   The joy of reading spiritual books: Getting lost in the wonder of prayer and divine presence, in God's presence as energy in every form and expression of the material world.

5.   The joy of sewing (yes, sewing, only discovered at the age of 76), cooking, gardening: New ventures with no goal except the fun and joy they offer me or others when shared.

6.   The joy of a home decorated for Christmas: Warm smells from the oven, the smell of spice in the air, and every corner of the house adorned in pine and red-and-green checkered ribbon.

7.   The joy of sitting with a loved one watching an extraordinary film: Drawn in together in a drama depicting human longing and the compassion shown to people who manifest a divine presence. An example would be the recent viewing of The Zoo Keeper's Wife, the true story of a Polish woman who saved Jews during the Holocaust by hiding them in her Warsaw zoo.

8.   The joy of cardio exercise: The sheer joy of muscles pressed to the max and a heart beating that wants to explode in your chest, the feel of blood coursing through your body with every pore of your skin offering droplets of water, as a way of cooling you off.

9.   The joy of savoring braised or roasted meats and caramelized roasted veggies: Kitchen smells and the natural sugars and fats of meats and vegetables coloring all a golden brown.

10. The joy of feeling good and looking well dressed: To recapture the pride of your mother or father when seeing you all spiffed up, except now it is you having the feeling of pride.

Yes, suns do exist. Note them and live in the bright light of them daily or at least weekly!

JOY IN ITS FULLNESS

Sustaining such levels, joy finds its success in dealing with stresses, as they occur and even before they occur, by maintaining daily ways of encountering joy as we have just seen. But this is not enough. Daily habitual contemplative practice grounds the believer firmly in his or her concrete living situation, moving them to the transcendent realm of the Cosmic Christ. The compassion that is experienced there is then applicable to the individual and expanded to others. Such compassionate care redounds in turn, to the believer and ultimately gives glory to God. And the cycle continues. However, rather than seeing it as circular, I like to think of it as a spiral that, like mattress springs of old, each deepening circle of the spring gets smaller and smaller in diameter until it is no longer the spring. Analogously, the individual becomes lost in God, and the fullness of joy has been received, experienced, and passed on to others.

THE BIRTH OF CONTEMPLATIVE ACTION AS COMPASSION

When compassion fills my heart,

free from all desire,

I sit quietly like the earth.

My silent cry echoes like thunder

throughout the universe.

– Rumi[174]

I continue to be struck by the insight that two things become evident when one is drawn into the divine presence through contemplation. The first is that you are *nothing* before the Presence, and this, the mystics call "wisdom." The second is that you are *everything,* and this they call "love." From this vantage point, love is not a muscle to be exercised and exerted in particular circumstances, as in "I will love her!" or "I will apologize to him for what I did." While the intention may well be there, the motivation or energy — no, let us call it what it is, the *grace* — comes from a much richer and deeper source. In contemplative prayer, the beholder is one with the creative, sustaining, redeeming source that we call God. It is a kind of cosmic energy flow. More on this cosmic energy later. Knowing you are nothing (no-thing) places you in a total stance of receiving what is being offered and humbled

---

[174] Narjis Pierre, "When Compassion Fills My Heart," Compassionate San Antonio, accessed April 20, 2017, http://sacompassionnet.org/poem-when-compassion-fills-my-heart/.

in the offering. There is no "I" and "you." There is only the gaze of union, the rapture of oneness. Teresa of Ávila calls it the "prayer of Union."[175]

It is out of such union that the grace and desire for compassion is born. The humbling empowerment shifts feeling one's "nothingness" to feeling one's "everything." The ego is diminished and with it the need to be right not wrong, control not be controlled, win and not lose. The embers of compassion burst into flame as the shift takes place, as contemplative prayer becomes contemplative action. Now all it takes is for the individual to see the pain of another to have his heart moved to compassion, to suffer with, as the derivation of the word implies. Born of compassion in the Presence, we become that very same compassion for others. Rohr would hold that,

> "It isn't enough to merely know that this wave is flowing through us; Spirit actually delights in it! The foundation of authentic Christian spirituality is not fear, but joy. Not hatred, but love. It's not error of God but actually participation in the very mystery of God."[176]

We know from scientific proof that such acts stimulate within the doer the release of substances within the pleasure centers of the brain. You might say we are wired for compassion and the joy that being compassionate brings. What brings a temporary end to such wiring and its wonderful effects is the return of self-interest and seeing the other as other. As this takes place, the existential experience of being "nothing and everything" is temporarily lost, and we are back in the ego game of winning, controlling, and being right. Things will not be set aright or the course of action redirected until the next session of contemplative prayer, when the right relationship with the divine and the human is reset.

MAKING GOLD OF BASE METALS

Alchemy was the medieval forerunner of modern chemistry. It was based on the supposed transformation of matter and concerned itself particularly with attempts to convert base metals into gold. It has come to

---

[175] "I still want to describe this prayer of quiet to you in the way that I have heard it explained and as the Lord has been pleased to teach it to me...This is a supernatural state and however hard we try, we cannot acquire it by ourselves...The faculties are stilled and have no wish to move, for any movement they make seems to hinder the soul from loving God. They are not completely lost, however, since two of them are free and they can realize in whose presence they are. It is the will that is captive now...The intellect tries to occupy itself with only one thing, and the memory has no desire to busy itself with more. They both see that this is the one thing necessary; anything else will cause them to be disturbed" (Chapter 31), https://www.catholicculture.org/culture/library/view.cfm?id=7725.

[176] Rohr, Trinity, Op. cit., 168.

imply a magical process of transformation. This book has been an attempt to see that transformation, not so much as magical, but no less real with the management of stress and the recapturing of joy that is available to every human being. Combining both the management and transformation contribute to creating the individual into the compassionate source from which they came, through which they move, and to transforming those who happen to be in their path that day. Raimon Panikkar says it most poignantly, "I am one with the source insofar as I act as a source by making everything I have received flow again — just like Jesus."[177] In his teaching and in our prayer, Jesus moves forward into this deepening spiral until we are nothing, and he is all in all. On our part, it takes surrendering, abandoning, throwing caution to the wind, all of which have been our traditional understanding of ascetical theology. When we no longer cling, when our joy becomes compassionate love toward all, the transformation — from the analogy of changing base metal to gold — has already taken place within us. Cynthia Bourgeault speaks of it as,

> "A kind of sacred alchemy. As we practice in daily life — in our acts of compassion, kindness, and self-emptying, both at the level of our doing and even more at the level of our being — something is catalyzed. Subtle qualities of divine love essential to the well-being of this planet are released through our actions and flow out into the world as miracle, healing, and hope."[178]

Yes, it is a kind of sacred alchemy not only in our doing, but at the level of our being as well. It is in this way, one person at a time, that the transformational flow out into the world has an impact on numerous others, who, in turn, impact others, and on and on it continues. It is far better than old alchemists could have hoped for in transforming a limited amount of matter into gold! This is not even to mention that you, as the receiver, have become the source, and the world is now afire with divine presence. It is the fullness of Jesus that he spoke of often, and it is the fullness to which he is calling us in the present.

TAKING THE PLUNGE

My friends and family have often called me a risk taker. However, I believe that there is a risk continuum from "foolhardy" to "calculated," and at anywhere on the continuum, there can be a bit of excitement and expectation. It is for this that I am often motivated to risk. As we conclude

[177] Raimon Panikkar, *Christophany: Fullness of Man,* (New York: Orbis Books, 2004), 116.
[178] Adapted from Cynthia Bourgeault, *The Wisdom Jesus: Transforming Heart and Mind—A New Perspective on Christ and His Message,* (Boston: Shambhala, 2008), 72-74.

this chapter and move on to our last, I want to encourage you, as the reader, to take the plunge into managing your stress, disposing yourself to the presence, and living out of that presence with love and compassion. With this "plunge," I leave you ten quotes regarding risk so you might see which fits you and your situation best.[179]

> "Whatever you can do, or dream you can, begin it. Boldness has genius, power and magic in it." — Goethe

> "Security is mostly a superstition. Life is either a daring adventure or nothing." — Helen Keller

> "It's not because things are difficult that we dare not venture. It's because we dare not venture that they are difficult." — Seneca

> "Only those who will risk going too far can possibly find out how far it is possible to go." — T.S. Eliot

> "What you have to do and the way you have to do it is incredibly simple. Whether you are willing to do it is another matter." — Peter Drucker

> "Go out on a limb. That's where the fruit is." — Jimmy Carter

> "I am always doing that which I cannot do, in order that I may learn how to do it." — Pablo Picasso

> "Life is being on the wire, everything else is just waiting." — Karl Wallenda

> "If things seem under control, you are just not going fast enough." — Mario Andretti

> "Don't be afraid to take a big step. You can't cross a chasm in two small jumps." — David Lloyd George

---

[179] Mitch Ditkoff, "50 Awesome Quotes on Risk Taking," The Blog, accessed April 21, 2017, last updated November 10, 2016, http://www.huffingtonpost.com/mitch-ditkoff/50-awesome-quotes-on-risk_b_2078573.html.

Possible Reflection Questions for Chapter 6: The Nature/Grace Reality in the Life of the Believer

- *What part do art, film, or music play in relieving your stress?*

- *What part do art, film, or music play in your experience of joy?*

- *On a scale of 1-10, with 10 being the highest, how egocentric would you say you are?*

- *What are your greatest obstacles in caring about others?*

Chapter 7:
Poised in a New Way:
Able to Handle Stress
Prayerfully, and Be There
for Others

Introduction

Something New

A New Context

Looking Forward

Parting Words

TWO ENEMIES OF CREATIVE WORK

Poet and author Wendell Berry says that the curse of creating is the struggle that the one creating experiences in shifting back-and-forth between despair and pride.[180] Both ends of the continuum are places one does not want to go. That creating is a struggle is known to anyone who has brought something new into being, from giving birth, sewing a handmade quilt, building a set of cabinets, planting a garden, preparing an original casserole, or creating a work of art. The work drains, fascinates, and engages us as it comes into being, bearing our own unique stamp. This work of book writing is no different. What kept my shoulder to the wheel was the desire not only to share experiences I have had regarding stress and how joy came out of it, but to delve into what, in each case, made the transition possible in myself as a youth and then as a middle school teacher who wanted to assist individuals in creating the same experience of joy within themselves. Yet, I realized from the beginning, it was not simply a human effort; rather, it involved God and the flow of grace, as very much a part of the process. Still, without the individual's participation, even God would not be able to accomplish the end alone! It would have to be a very real partnership.

This final chapter will hopefully be a very practical one: one where lessons understood (covered in Chapters 1 through 6) could become lessons applied (Chapter 7) and eventually, fruits acquired through regular practice. If that were to come to pass, the purpose of this work will have been achieved.

CHAPTER FORMAT

I thought it helpful to have the very title of the chapter lay out the format we would be following in order to make the application of what has been presented clear and easy to use. Thus, we begin by suggesting that the preceding chapters have helped us to be "Poised in a New Way" regarding the nature and management of stress, and "Poised in a New Way" in understanding the role that contemplation can play, not only in stress reduction, but more importantly, in creating the condition for grace to flow and to have joy be the culminating experience. The more both management and presence are practiced, the more the joy would become a lived and on-going experience. And even when joy was not being experienced, but no less desired, there would be concrete tools at hand to make a difference. To live out of this new paradigm would, however, require a shift in our normal way of solving our stress.

---

[180] Maria Popova, "Wendell Berry on Solitude and Why Pride and Despair Are Two Great Enemies of Creative Work," *Two-Handed Warriors*, January 4, 2015, accessed April 25, 2017, http://garydavidstratton.com/2015/01/04/wendell-berry-on-solitude-and-why-pride-and-despair-are-the-two-great-enemies-of-creative-work/.

A NECESSARY PARADIGM SHIFT

Thomas Koon speaks of a "paradigm shift" or what religion would call a "major conversion." Truth and evidence have little to do with any shift in these realms. They will remain as a deposit of what you believe and what you bring to it. We are so tied to our own positions that it is difficult to see past them. If you cannot detach from your own ideas, the ego becomes detached and running on its own limitations. The Kuhn Cycle is a simple cycle of progress described by Kuhn in 1962 in his foundational work entitled, *The Structure of Scientific Revolutions.*[181] The author challenges the conception of science, which states that all things are a steady progression of the simple accumulation of new ideas. Kuhn shows that such a viewpoint is wrong. To the contrary, science advances most by periodic explosions of new knowledge, each revolution being triggered by the introduction of a new way of thinking that is so large that it must be called a new paradigm. It is from Kuhn's work that the popular terms like "paradigm" and "paradigm shift" have come.

The Kuhn Cycle consists of the five steps, as shown in Figure 12. Kuhn's hypothesis is that great progress comes from revolutionary breakthroughs and has an equivalent in the life sciences. Richard Rohr has applied the breakthroughs to spiritual transformation as well.[182]

---

[181] "The Kuhn Cycle," thwink.org, accessed April 24, 2017, http://www.thwink.org/sustain/glossary/KuhnCycle.htm.

[182] *Trinity: The Soul of Creation,* with Richard Rohr, Cynthia Bourgeault, and Wm Paul Young, Session 2 (April 6-8, 2017), http://cac.org/trinity-webcast/.

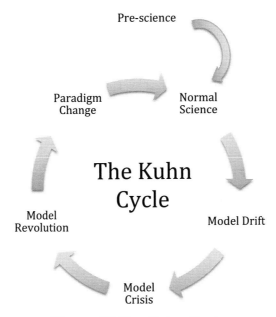

Figure 12 The Kuhn Cycle

In "The Kuhn Cycle," we see how the process proceeds in five stages: (1) What is Normally Known; to a (2) Drift in what is known; to a (3) Crisis in what is known; to a (4) Revolution in what is known; to a (5) Paradigm Change regarding what is known. "Drift" gets you to let go a bit from the usual way of solving a challenge. "Crisis" serves as the motivation to do something about it. "Revolution" creates the upset and generates solutions. What emerges is the new way of doing things, the new "Paradigm Change." For us, it is not about logic or easy answers. Real change, lasting change, is about the drift and crisis that stress produces and the revolution and change that grace effects. Thus, we find in the spiritual life that what first appears, as a huge negative becomes, quite surprisingly, the cusp of change. Of course for Christians, the reality is experienced in the words of St. Paul where he hears from the Lord,

> " 'My grace is sufficient for you, for power is perfected in weakness.' Most gladly, therefore, I will rather boast about my weaknesses, so that the power of Christ may dwell in me. Therefore, I am well content with weaknesses, with insults, with distresses, with persecutions, with difficulties, for Christ's sake; for when I am weak, then I am strong."[183]

---

[183] 2 Corinthians 12:9–11, (New American Standard Bible).

BEHOLD, I AM DOING SOMETHING NEW

"See, I am doing a new thing!

Now it springs up; do you not perceive it?

I am making a way in the wilderness

and streams in the wasteland."[184]

In the 43rd Chapter of Isaiah, the prophet presents a series of arguments in order to assure the Israelites that they will be restored, no matter how great their turning from God has been. The restoration will be new and unprecedented, and the "springing forth" elicits the silent, though gradual growth of events that are to take place. The events will take place where the Israelites find themselves in the moment, just as their forbearers found themselves in the wilderness between the Red Sea and the Promised Land. And just as a way was opened for their ancestors, so will a way be opened for them again in the wilderness of the entire world, and the prophecy will again be fulfilled.

OLD WAY —> NEW WAY

It is easy to understand the "Old Way," that is, how we have managed or not managed stress and how we have been able or unable to pray. In applying what has been learned in previous chapters of the present work, a "New Way" has hopefully emerged. Contrasting the two can help us move to the new paradigm. So let us begin our considerations of the "Old" and "New."

OLD WAY —> NEW WAY OF "HANDLING STRESS"

For me, over the years, my Old Way has been the exercise of sheer willpower, grinning and bearing it, gritting my teeth…you know the routine. At other times, I have simply left the scene, if it was an employee that I was stressing over, for example. However, if it was a superior, and I just could not leave the scene gracefully, I would revert to the willpower technique just mentioned. Unfortunately, it is a great way to wear down your teeth and eventually have need of a mouth guard for sleeping. Other avenues I used, included thinking of other things, minimizing the stress by comparing it to

---

[184] Isaiah 43:15, (New International Version).

larger stresses I have been through, picturing the individual in a humorous way (so I would not have to take them seriously), or letting off steam with a friend. In looking at these as a whole, they do not seem very effective, long lasting, or creative to the relationships. More to the heart of the matter, they took a toll on blood pressure, acid stomach, or different levels of psychological stress.

As they say, "having lived and learned" and having the psychological resources, I am now able to come to the situation armed with tools that work much more effectively. I am able to note that I am stressed, determine how stressed I really am, use specific tools for each of the three stress levels covered in preceding chapters, depending on whether I am very stressed, somewhat stressed, or already in a state of joy. The application of specific tools to specific levels of stress changes everything in terms of effectiveness, at least for a start. With the gaining of a certain level of equanimity, I can also then dispose myself to contemplative prayer and be present to the Presence.

With a sense of calm, I am now able to open myself in surrender and vulnerability in order to experience a oneness that is both healing and generative. Let us not forget the alternative of a "joy jolt," if stress levels are low. Here, you may remember, we simply go to an image, piece of music, work of art, or project accomplished, and take delight in it. For me, it may be looking at the car I just washed, recalling an excellent article I have recently read, simply warming my face in the sun, or striking a Yoga pose. A final enhancement technique I employ is to have several easy-to-do activities at the ready, so every day you can do at least one or use one when you need a break from an energy-sapping project in which you are involved. For me, that may be watching an 18-minute TED Talk, listening to *The Moth* (real life audio clips on Public Radio), checking out an online recipe, or just surfing the internet regarding an interesting topic. The only caution is that any one of these should serve as a 10- or 15-minute break from the routine or a demanding job you are doing.

OLD WAY —> NEW WAY FOR *"PRAYERFULLY..."*

The Old Way for me amounted to praying in exasperation. This included crying out to God, "Why me Lord, why now?" — or something akin to St. Teresa's response to God when her wagon got caught in the Castilian mud, and she cried out, "Lord, if this is the way you treat your friends, it's no wonder you have so few of them!" A second line of defense that involved prayer would include specific prayers in times of distress. In this regard, even with the best of intentions, the stress loomed too strong, and the verbal prayers were not an even match over so powerful a force.

The New Way of prayer may be either contemplation or meditation, if the latter is a practice for you. What is different here is that you are dealing directly with some of the stress, and there is a greater ability to go deeper into communion with God. Having a specific setting (room, chair, candle, icon, etc.), a specific time of day (mornings before others are stirring), and a routine (mantra, synchronization to breathing, letting go, and resting in God) all contribute to creating the possibility of a more effective communion with God. Developing a habit of doing this 10–20 minutes a day adds to the ease of doing it. At times, I will bring in what I call "flavor-oids," items that add to the delight of the moment, things such as a steaming cup of coffee, a scented candle, wistful music, or a burning a stick of incense. It is interesting how the Church has used some of these within the service and after Mass — serving coffee, for example. Olfactory senses are very powerful inasmuch as they go right to the brain without any mental processing, and when smelled, they recall delightful experiences, past and present. As we have already noted, if it is too difficult to remain in contemplative presence because of distractions and compulsive thinking, feel free to move to meditation and image creation for a rich dialog with the Divine.

OLD WAY —> NEW WAY FOR *"BEING THERE..."*

"Be Here Now" is a phrase used often in the spirituality literature. It is a simple way of inviting one into letting go of concerns and thinking of all kinds — just being, with nothing added.[185] When you become truly present, you will have all you need to know, for your mind is what keeps you away from and out of the present. It is interesting how the mind can both repackage the past and be anxious of the future, but it can't be in the present! Not only then, is the mind the primary thing keeping you out of the present, more importantly, it is keeping you away from what is being revealed there. It takes putting the mind into the heart by using simple techniques or tools to disengage it. To live in this way — out of your heart — is a very powerful experience. We know that people can die from a broken heart. In this regard, we often speak of head space, heart space, and body space. All three elements need to be tended for us to be present. No, your mind is not to be thrown out. You just need to let go of its monkey-mind tendency and be totally available to the present moment. While there is cortical activity, there is no cognitive activity; there is just awareness.

---

[185] *Be Here Now,* as a phrase, began as the title of a 1971 book on spirituality, yoga, and meditation by the Western-born yogi and spiritual teacher Ram Dass (born Richard Alpert).

Scattered and compulsive thinking are clearly inhibiters to being in the present, and with this sort of thinking, you will inevitably find yourself *at the effect* of all the mental activity in your head, rather than at the calm you are seeking. Stressful thoughts, daydreaming, thoughts involving the making of plans, or just wistful thoughts to keep you from boredom or monotony, all will put you *at their effect* and keep you out of what the present moment may be offering. On the other hand, being *at the cause* of your thoughts, seen as your efforts of having no thoughts or managing thinking, will be your part in opening up the pulsating presence. When such a state is achieved, which was the topic of Chapter 4, you can relax into the present and have it reveal its treasures of peace, tranquility, and spaciousness.

The New Way of "Being There" that has you into the shift to no thinking will necessitate a kind of death to the ego and all those things that are seemingly so important to its existence. It will also include giving up the tendency of dualistic thinking, where you are judging others, situations, or things as either good or bad, in or out, acceptable or not. One final thing that will be surrendered is having *to do something* as a way of "being there." There is nothing to do that can be richer or more effective than what the present moment has to offer the person who comes to it with an open and loving heart. Most times, seven to 10 repetitions of deep breathing are all I need to clear my head, calm my nerves, and put me headlong into the redeeming present.

OLD WAY —> NEW WAY
"FOR OTHERS"

Jim Finley, noted psychologist and spiritual writer, states that through contemplative prayer we, "follow the saints on the path of compassionate love that heals the roots of suffering [and stress] that have found their way into our minds and hearts."[186]

Loving others in the Old Way was like going to boot camp and preparing for battle. It would be as if love were a muscle that needed to be toned and then exercised by the sheer power of our wills and, having done so, would get us to the place where, with gritted teeth and clenched jaw, we would be able to say, "I *will* love, him/her! I *will* forgive him/her!"

To be there "For Others" in the New Way is to live out of contemplative presence, which is a rare ability and a gift from God. Doing so, with a heart renewed, you will surprise yourself at how far you will go to reach out and love

---

[186] The above mentioned is number 5 of Jim Finley's 7 principles, *Transforming Trauma: Exploring the Spiritual Dimensions of Healing*, Manuscript, Gerry May Shalem Seminar, April 24-25, 2015.

others. Lucien Desis, a church composer of the 1970's, composed a beautiful hymn on this very topic, the refrain of which was, "Grant to us, O Lord, a heart renewed. Recreate in us your own spirit, Lord."[187] Of course, the truth is that it is *not* you. The truth is you have, through contemplative presence, become the very presence of God to others and whatever acts of love, forgiveness, or compassion you find yourself performing, you know it is by the very grace of God through which you are acting. Eventually friends, neighbors, or family members will notice the difference and ask, "What happened to you!" The simple answer is that you have gotten into the flow of God's love and are now able to live buoyed up by it. There is no longer any effort needed to swim. You are literally being carried by the flow and moving gently down river. What an extraordinary state of being!

JUST ENOUGH CUSHION SITTING

Serious advocates of sitting-in-silence refer to their devoted time to the presence as "cushion sitting." I, along with Thomas Keating and the Centering Prayer School that he and others have developed, would suggest two 20-minute sessions a day — one in the morning and one in the evening. Recommendations for the length and number of sessions are given as a guide, and in this regard "more may not be better." Spending large amounts of time may become, like drugs, a way of escaping reality. To the question of why twice a day for 20 minutes and not one longer period Keating responds,

> "Twice a day keeps you closer to the reservoir of silence. If you get too far away from the reservoir, it is like being on the end of the water line after everybody has taken what they want from the reservoir. When you turn on the faucet, you only get a few drops. To prevent that from happening, keep the pressure up. You need to keep filling your reservoir until you eventually strike an artesian well. Then the water is always flowing."[188]

This is to say that you do not need to spend hours sitting in prayer for the proper disposition and flow of grace to take place. It is developing a sense of inner silence, which becomes the source of a wellspring within you.

Sufficient is the time spent in contemplative prayer when it animates the contemplative action for your day. For starters, it may be helpful not to separate prayer and action into two distinct activities. Here I mean that, freed

[187] Lucien Deiss, CSSp, "Grant to Us O Lord," Youtube, February 22, 2015, accessed April 25, 2017, https://www.youtube.com/watch?v=PxkTLzgNZsw.
[188] Thomas Keating, *Open Mind, Open Heart: The Contemplative Dimension of the Gospel*, (New York: Continuum International Publishing Group, 2006), 58.

up from constraints of stress, the experience of the divine, no matter how long it is, will change your perspective in the way you see things in your environment. However the experience is described — be it as rest, silence, tranquility, bondedness, warmth, or love — it will of necessity dispose your heart, as you transition from the silence to your world of noise and responsibility. What will arise, as you gently reenter your world of activity, is the question of how you can move and relate, as God has moved and related with you in the silence. What a powerful force contemplation would have become in such applications!

To sum up the prayer-action continuum, when you enter contemplation and have rid yourself of stress, thinking, and distractions, you float for a time in the timeless, endless heart of God. And it is precisely there that you live for a time in an unconstrained and timeless synchrony. It is this "abiding" — to use Jesus' word — in which you become part of an extraordinary newness. So it is not so much a having-to-change-your-old-self; it is more that you are able to trust and draw on the instantaneous life-giving presence to which you have been party. Consequently, you now move into each situation of the day and see what is needed or called for, and you make it support a disinterested commitment to work on its behalf.

You do not need to sit on your cushion 10 hours a day. We have only to look at the tireless dedication of people who are committed to pray like Mother Theresa, Desmond Tutu, or Martin Luther King and their caring for the world to see the impact that such unified prayer and action can have. No question about it, we are co-creators within the divine heart of God, revealing more and more dimensions of divine love in the world in which we live.

A final note in this regard: even in the midst of the violence and atrocities we may be experiencing both in our nation and the world at any given time, we are better able to enter those places in conscious service, based on the trust that is ours from the presence. Within that trust, we will have learned a way to determine what needs to be done. In our little corner of the world, our choice of right actions on behalf of justice will be our contribution to the very revelation of the Divine Heart. That is the ultimate union of contemplative prayer and contemplative action!

A HEART RENEWED, RECREATED

Compassion is a feeling or emotion that helps move individuals toward caring for others. It surfaces from coming to understand that we are all in some way connected. Our earliest experiences of compassion are learned as children, and as adults they may need to be relearned, for in adulthood, the survival of the ego tends to take center stage. In the West, such relearning and the experience of being connected to all that lives can be relearned through contemplative prayer, where the unitive experience is truly that — a union with all that is — and thus acting lovingly and compassionately is the natural outcome of such an experienced presence. The Dalai Lama speaks of compassion as,

> "The wish that others be free of suffering. It is by means of compassion that we aspire to attain enlightenment. It is compassion that inspires us to engage in the virtuous practices that lead to Buddhahood. We must therefore devote ourselves to developing compassion."[189]

The Four Noble Truths of Buddhism are spoken of as the plan for dealing with the suffering we all experience, be it physical, mental, or spiritual and how the Truths help us to gain compassion.[190]

Cynthia Bourgeault teaches beautifully on this new way of being there for others. She writes, "When our hearts are gentled and single, when we've tamed the animal instincts, we become peacemakers."[191] We no longer need to come from our own power and strength and dividing the world into good and bad guys, those who belong and those who do not, winners and losers.[192] "When our peace and grounding come from a deeper presence to the divine," she continues, "an inner peaceableness flows into the outer world as harmony and compassion. This is what we mean by contemplative engagement."[193] It is clearly action in the world and action grounded in divine grace. She would claim that, "Only from the unified perception of the heart

---

[189] The Dalai Lama, *An Open Heart: Practicing Compassion in Everyday Life,* (Little, Brown and Co., 2001), 91.

[190] The First Truth identifies the presence of suffering. The Second Truth attempts to understand the cause of suffering. Buddhism holds that it is desire and ignorance that lies at the root of all suffering. Desire is the craving of pleasure, material goods, and immortality, all of which are wants that can never be satisfied. Because they are not achievable, desiring any one of them can only bring about suffering. Ignorance, in contrast, relates to not seeing the world as it actually is. Without the capacity for mental concentration and insight, a person's mind is left undeveloped, unable to grasp the true nature of things. All of the vices, e.g. greed, envy, hatred and anger, flow from this ignorance. The Third Noble Truth, the truth regarding the end of suffering, can either mean the end of suffering on earth or, in the spiritual life, by achieving Nirvana. In achieving Nirvana, a transcendent state that is free of suffering, spiritual enlightenment is reached. Finally, the Fourth Noble truth charts the method for attaining the end of suffering. http://www.pbs.org/edens/thailand/buddhism.htm.

[191] Cynthia Bourgeault, "The Beatitudes, Be Peaceable, Be Free," April 21, 2017, accessed April 29, 2017, https://cac.org/be-peaceable-be-free-2017-04-21/.

[192] What comes to mind is the resoluteness of Pope Francis in saying how he was going to meet with President Donald Trump. While he will not try to convince him to ease his policies on immigration and the environment, he said he is more concerned with finding areas where the two might agree in order to work more effectively towards peace. http://www.washingtonexaminer.com/pope-on-meeting-with-trump-i-never-make-a-judgement-about-a-person-without-hearing-him-out/article/2623043.

[193] Ibid.

can we discern what action is required of us to lovingly and effectively serve our hurting planet."[194] The recreated heart is a radical transformation of a new heart from the old heart. It is open, non-egoic, trusting, risking, and willing to dive headlong into the flow of the river. In the end, what our own participation contributes to is the decrease of violent interactions and egocentric grasping that is so much of our world culture today. This teaching has a ring to it that is very similar to the teachings of all the great religious leaders of our world today and resonates with the ancient traditions of the Christian mystics as well.

THE ROLES WE PLAY AND WHERE THEY FIT

We need to look at the roles we have played in the past, are playing now, and could be playing in the future. Distinguishing among them can open new possibilities for us in a creative and life-giving way. For example, as a spouse before your children were born, how were you as a nurturing and forgiving person? How did that role evolve when you became a parent to a toddler? To a teenager? To your child as a young adult? How did it evolve as a Little League coach? As a volunteer in your parish? And so the applications go on and on. What is important to note is that each prior role you play can prepare you for what has not yet been defined, and what emerges is built on the template of the prior iteration. Where the excitement might come is standing in the present and, buoyed up by the flow of the river, asking, what is the nudge of grace you may be feeling for what may be awakening within you? What are the possibilities? What is emerging? Clearly then, the emerging roles can relate to your profession, family situation, or your relationship to the world-at-large.

The infighting in the Vatican never seemed to get to Pope Francis. When reporters asked about it and raised other stresses of his job, his response was a shrug of the shoulders and a lighthearted response of, "I am not on tranquilizers." He admitted that indeed, there is corruption within the Vatican Curia, and assured them, "But I am at peace."[195]

---

[194] Ibid.

[195] "Pope Francis reveals how he shrugs off stress: I'm not on tranquilizers," The Guardian, accessed April 29, 2017, https://www.theguardian.com/world/2017/feb/09/pope-francis-reveals-how-he-shrugs-off-stress-im-not-on-tranquilisers.

GAINING A SENSE OF SELF
AND GIVING IT AWAY

We live our lives in a steady stream of consciousness, which is a continual flow of ideas, images, and feelings.[196] And at every moment, we tend to cling to these thoughts and sensations so much so that it feels as if we do not have the idea, but that the idea has us! We do not have the feeling; the feeling has us. We can spend a lifetime trying to discover who this "I" really is. Is it the one having these passing feelings and thoughts or is there another "I" behind my thoughts and feelings? The fixed point that watches things pass through me — that is the real me. Contemplative prayer helps us to understand how to abide in this deepest place and to abide there in peace. We have to find a way to get beyond our self-image and our ideas about who we are. We have to discover the face that we already had before we were born, who we were in God all along — before we did anything right or wrong. This is the first goal of contemplation. This is the "I" that is capable of union with God.

Here is an exercise that some find helpful. Imagine a river or stream. You are sitting on the bank of this river, where boats and ships are sailing past. While the stream flows past your inner eye, I would ask you to name each one of the "vessels" or thoughts floating by. For example, one of the boats could be called "my anxiety about tomorrow." Or along comes the ship "objections to my spouse" or "I don't do that well." Every judgment that passes by you is one of these boats. Take the time to give each one of them a name, and then *let it move on*. For some people, this is a very difficult exercise to perform because we are used to jumping aboard our boats immediately and in doing so, we give them gas! As soon as we take a boat to ourselves and identify with it, it seems to pick up its own energy. We have to practice un-possessing, letting go, detaching from our thoughts and feelings, or they will surely drive us.

Some of the boats to which we are accustomed, and on which we jump aboard readily, have passed us by only with heroic efforts on our part to let them do so. However, they will immediately make a U-turn and head back upstream to return, trying to catch our attention again and again. Some people feel the need to torpedo such boats. But you must not attack, hate, or condemn any idea or thought; to do so would merely be your perfectionistic ego trying to "win." If we learn to handle our own souls tenderly and lovingly, then we will be able to carry this same loving wisdom into our other relationships. A thousand seeming "distractions" are now a thousand opportunities to choose God instead. So there is no reason to label a distraction as bad or eschewed. Why did not someone tell me that as a novice so many years ago!

[196] Antonio Damasio, "The Quest to Understand Consciousness," TED Talk, March 2011, accessed April 29, 2017, https://www.ted.com/talks/antonio_damasio_the_quest_to_understand_consciousness.

Using the tools we have considered, we might ask, "Who or what is the self that has been calmed of stress, and is ready to enter contemplative prayer?" Antonio Damasio, a well-known researcher in the field of neuroscience, speaks of waking from sleep each morning and regaining consciousness and asks just what is it that you regain each morning.[197] What it is is the recovery of a sense that we are (existence) and a sense of who we are (identity). Without this astonishing capability, we would never know pain, nor for that matter, joy. He quotes Scott Fitzgerald, who quipped, "He who invented consciousness would have a lot to be blamed for." But it is not all bad; without consciousness, we would also have no access to the possibility of transcendence and the experience of joy. Stress and joy are two sides of a single coin. Damasio makes a great case of how the brain is able to create consciousness and attempts to demonstrate that fact quite compellingly.[198] It is this sense of being and of being me that I am able to bring to the table of contemplation only to give it up, free myself from it, for a deeper, richer sense of being and self, namely being *in* God and being *for* others. And it is precisely in this experience within the presence that I become all God has destined me to be. The reward? The payoff? Joy unending!

TIME UNDER THE WATER SPRINKLER

When I recall the joy of my childhood, it takes me back to the age of four or five and all of us children in the heat of summer, donned simply in our underwear, jumping and giggling in the 20 minutes we were allotted under the sprinkler. Not wasting water was a creed we lived by as members of an immigrant urban family. At 15 minutes would come the ominous cry of my mother, "Five minutes to go!" At that point the giggling would become fever-pitched screaming, the jumping and trouncing would become more animated, and it was as if we were trying to get all the joy we could out of the water flow, knowing it would soon be turned off. That vivid childhood image taught me that living in the grace of the present moment was all you needed. Savoring it, resting, and delighting within it was all it took. Anything could become a 20-minute sprinkler experience. It seems that as children we were able to do this until, that is, we were taught not to trust the moment, much less to live it with wild abandon. If God is a good God all the time — as say my mother, father, or favorite teacher was good — we can live in the grace of one day, risking and playfully delighting in what we have. Joy is in the presence of God, and it is right here in the grace of this one-day, and God

---

[197] Ibid.
[198] Ibid.

does not have his hand on the faucet ready to turn off the water. When joy is not experienced, it is not because the spark of joy cannot be rekindled, but it is more that stress has reduced it to an ember so much so that it isn't even felt. Living inside the grace of the day, there is always enough to rekindle the spark and have it blaze. We were designed to be children in relationship with a loving God and in relationship with those we love.

THE PROMISE

In workshops, they call them objectives. In consultations or deal-making meetings, they call them deliverables. In spirituality, they are called functions. Yet, no matter what they are called, they are the fruits of planning on the part of those who invested themselves in the task of producing an improved outcome. This book has attempted to offer deeper, more lasting ways for managing your daily stress that, when developed, can offer you a way inward to the joy that lies within you. In this concluding chapter, and with the appendices offered, the reader will hopefully come away with a handy way for both understanding the stresses in life and having a cadre of practical ways to contact that deeper inner experience of joy.

JOY AT THE READY

Armed with tools for stress reduction and contemplative prayer, you will find yourself going from a level of edginess to boundless compassion for others. As you continue to use the tools of both the psychological and spiritual disciplines, it will become easier and more a lifestyle. You and others will begin to notice the change. Dare we say that stress then, is an opportunity that we had not before realized? Can stress and joy in fact be bedfellows? The inner strength that comes from presence can meet the challenge of stress, once the stress has been managed enough to free the mind to sit in stillness in order to simply receive. It is only in recent times that the studies in neuropsychology and spirituality have come together to offer believers new avenues of growth and a deepening life of joy at-the-ready.

THE MEETING OF STRESS AND TRUE JOY

Francis told his friars that their vocation in life was to serve as God's minstrels, that is, "To move people's hearts and lift them up to spiritual joy."[199] They needed no other justification for their life of ministry. An incident involving Francis and Bro. Leo on the road from Perugia to Assisi makes the point.

In the bitter cold, Francis calls out to Bro. Leo five times, telling him what perfect joy was not,

> "Brother Leo, even if a Friar Minor gives sight to the blind, heals the paralyzed, drives out devils, gives hearing back to the deaf, makes the lame walk, and restores speech to the dumb, and what is more brings back to life a man who has been dead four days, write that perfect joy is not in that."

After two miles of this walking conversation on the subject, Bro. Leo cries out, "Father, I beg you in God's name to tell me where perfect joy is then to be found?" His reply is both cryptic and profound,

> "When we come to the Portiuncula, soaked by the rain and frozen by the cold, all soiled with mud and suffering from hunger, and we ring at the gate of our friary and the brother porter comes and says angrily: 'Who are you?' and we say: 'We are two of your brothers.' And he contradicts us, saying, 'You are not telling the truth. Rather you are two rascals who go around deceiving people and stealing what they give to the poor. Go away!' and he does not open for us, but makes us stand outside in the snow and rain, cold and hungry until night falls — then if we endure all of those insults and cruel rebuffs patiently, without being troubled and without complaining, and if we reflect humbly and lovingly that the porter really knows us. Oh, Brother Leo, write that perfect joy is to be found there!"

But it doesn't end there. Francis continues,

> "And if we continue to knock and the porter comes out in anger, and drives us away with curses and hard blows saying 'Get away from here! Who do you think you are?' and if we bear it patiently and take the insults with joy and love in our

---

[199] St. Francis of Assisi, *Francis of Assisi - Early Documents*, vol. 2, (Hyde Park: New City Press, 2000), 186.

hearts. Oh, Brother Leo, write down that this is perfect joy!...
And now hear the conclusion: Above all the graces and gifts
of the Holy Spirit which Christ gives to his friends is that of
conquering oneself and willingly enduring sufferings, insults,
humiliations, and hardships for the love of Christ."[200]

While managing stress is important for disposing ourselves to God's
presence, it's very experience, even before it is "managed," according to
Francis can be a moment of blessing and an occasion for gratitude.

A DECISION TO BE MADE

Evangelist Billy Graham tells the story of an Eskimo fisherman who
came to town every Saturday afternoon. He always brought his two dogs
with him. One was white, and the other was black. He had taught them to
fight, on command. Every Saturday afternoon in the town square, the people
would gather, and these two dogs would fight, and the fisherman would take
bets. On one Saturday, the black dog would win; another Saturday the white
dog would win, but the fisherman always won! His friends began to ask him
how he did it. He quietly whispered to him, "I starve one and feed the other.
The one I feed always wins because he is stronger." And so it is with joy as a
"winner." There is a fundamental decision that needs to be made: to starve the
stress and feed the joy for it to flow through contemplative prayer, or to feed
the stress and starve yourself of the Presence.

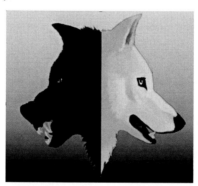

Figure 13 The One I Feed [201]

---

[200] St. Francis of Assisi, ed Marion A. Habig, *St. Francis of Assisi: Omnibus of the Sources*,
(Franciscan Herald Press: 1973), 1318–1320.
[201] http://www.oneyoufeed.net/wp-content/uploads/2014/01/TOYF_Avatar-smaller-file-size-
1000x1000.jpg

JOY IN ROUGH TIMES

Let us admit it: very often we act with a sense of entitlement that everything in our lives run smoothly and, only then, can we be joyful. Contrary to that fact, life is seldom or rarely okay for us or our loved ones. It is just not the way the world seems to run. Yet, is not joy necessary even in those circumstances, which are the norm of everyone's life? Wendell Berry's writings are filled with what he once described as, "A free nonhuman joy in the world." He tells of a time when he was weighed down with worry and stress, and at a moment, he caught sight of a Great Blue Heron making its stately descent. Without warning, the elegant bird turned backward in midair, did a loop-the-loop, and flew out of Berry's sight. His mood turned from heaviness to delight. "I don't see many Great Blue Herons, but if I become truly aware of the creatures around me, big and small, their approach to life often brings me joy even in the darkest of times."[202]

Then there is Francis of Assisi, who was experiencing great pain in going blind. Yet, in this pool of pain, he composed his beautiful *Canticle of the Sun.*[203] In it, he takes great joy in the sun, moon, stars, wind, water, and fire, which he describes as "beautiful and playful and robust and strong." Francis' Canticle is like a checklist of things that can bring us joy in hard times. We might go over that checklist when our spirits are down. Yes, there is always joy available in rough times. All it takes is noticing and connecting!

THE WRITING OF THIS BOOK

As I mentioned at the opening of this chapter, Wendell Berry speaks of pride and despair as two sides of a single coin, claiming that both are equally culpable in poisoning creative work and pushing us toward loneliness rather than toward the sharing of values, which the art calls forth. Despair seems to come of taking too little responsibility, whereas pride is concerned with taking too much of it. This work has been built on deep questions I have had about the interplay of joy and stress. It was studied in the practical living out of my role as Spiritual Integrator at St. Luke's Institute, and it was applied within weekend and seven-day retreat settings, thus bringing the question full circle from head to heart to application in the lives of clergy and religious in residential care, as well as religious and laity in retreat settings. It is my hope that for you, good work has been borne of the endeavor of writing this book. I conclude with the words of Berry,

---

[202] Maria Popova, "A Benediction on the World: Wendall Barry on Creaturely Joy," Brainpickings, https://www.brainpickings.org/2016/08/02/wendell-berry-great-blue-heron/.

[203] "Saint Francis of Assisi," The Humane Society of the United States, accessed May 1, 2017, http://www.humanesociety.org/about/departments/faith/francis_files/st_francis_of_assisi.html?credit=blog_post_032113_id4235?referrer=https://www.google.com/.

"True solitude is found in the wild places, where one is without human obligation. One's inner voices become audible. One feels the attraction of one's most intimate sources. In consequence, one responds more clearly to other lives. The more coherent one becomes within oneself as a creature, the more fully one enters into the communion of all creatures."[204]

STAYING IN TOUCH

Over the years, participants of the retreats and days of recollection I have led, as well as readers of my BlogSpot, Facebook page, and Mepkin Abbey webpage, have emailed or texted me with questions or insights to share regarding how contemplative prayer has impacted their daily lives. I am always open to such communications and do make time to respond to them in a timely fashion. It is part of a new effort in using social media as a way to spread the good news of the Gospel.

The easiest way to connect is by simply Googling *Father Nicholas Amato* into your browser, and all the available links for my BlogSpot, Facebook page, Twitter account, and Mepkin Trappist Abbey site will be offered. My email address is: fathernicholasamato@gmail.com.

A dear friend of many years was slowing dying from emphysema. In her final days, she said to me, "Nicholas, I will save you a seat!" In recapturing the joy beneath your stress, I would claim that we are already there in heaven. To simply draw each other into the presence, in that case, would be enough.

Possible Reflection Questions for Chapter 7: Poised in a New Way: Able to Handle Stress Prayerfully, and Be There for Others

---

    ❧   *What might be a "New Way" for you to handle stress?*

    ❧   *What might be a "New Way" for you to pray?*

    ❧   *What might be a "New Way" for you to be there for others?*

---

[204] Maria Popova, "Wendall Berry on Solitude and Why Pride and Despair Are the Two Great Enemies of Creative Work," Brainpickings, https://www.brainpickings.org/2014/12/17/wendell-berry-pride-despair-solitude/.

Appendices

Author's Note: The following appendices are offered as resources to move you as the reader...

- From reading of the book
- To reflecting on the questions after each chapter
- To implementing the instruction and reflections into your lifestyle.

Appendix A: Concerning Stress

SYMPTOMS OF STRESS

(Source: Gillian Bethel, From Stress to Joy, (Roseville: Amazing Facts, Inc., 2004), 317.)

PHYSICAL

- Frequent nervous "tics" or muscle spasms
- Frequent infections and viruses
- Dry mouth
- Stiffness, tension, and pain of neck, back, and joints
- Frequent abdominal pain
- Frequent indigestion, diarrhea, or constipation
- Itchy skin
- Arms crossed or fists clenched while conversing
- Clutching the steering wheel in traffic
- Easily startled
- Frequent headaches
- Frequent insomnia, fatigue, loss of appetite

PSYCHOLOGICAL

- Frequent feelings of panic and/or not being in control
- Frequent depression for no apparent reason
- Difficulty concentrating on the simplest tasks
- Frequent impatience
- Frequent forgetfulness
- Sudden emotional outbursts and crying spells
- Frequent worrying or feeling trapped by circumstances
- Frequent mood swings
- Frequent irritation over small difficulties
- Routine tasks become nearly unbearable to accomplish
- Frequent boredom and/or need for excitement/escapism
- Increased use of coping mechanisms: alcohol, caffeinated drinks, smoking, drug taking, eating, sleeping, etc.

HOW TO NAME STRESSORS

- Listening to what trusted friends notice that may be stressing you

- Listening to what a counselor or spiritual director mentions that may be stressing you

- Naming stressors for yourself

THREE LEVELS OF STRESS

(Source: Laurel Mellin, Wired for Joy: A Revolutionary Method for Creating Happiness from Within, (New York, Hays House, 2010), 139-56.)

- **State 1:** You're in the flow and your whole brain is in balance (Use of the Sanctuary Tool)

- **State 3:** You're a little stressed and emotions are ramping up, particularly negative ones (Use of the Emotional Housecleaning Tool)

- **State 5:** You're stressed out and over the top (Use of the Damage Control Tool)

TIPS TO REDUCE STRESS

(Source: Deanne Alban, "12 Effects of Chronic Stress on Your Brain," Be Brain Fit, accessed December 7, 2016, https://bebrainfit.com/effects-chronic-stress-brain/.)

- Eat a diet high in antioxidant-rich foods like fruit, vegetables, dark chocolate, and green tea

- Get daily physical exercise

- Begin a daily meditation practice. Meditation not only reduces stress, it's a proven way to keep your brain young. Meditation is also the best tool for learning how to master your thoughts. Stress does not come from events in your life as much as it comes from your thoughts — your automatic negative reactions and cognitive distortions — about these events

- Try mind-body relaxation techniques

- Look into taking an herbal remedy

QUESTIONS TO RESPOND TO:

- What are people, whose word I trust, telling me?

- How's it going with God?

- What are the surprises in my prayer life and noticings this past month?

- What are the resistances in my prayer life and noticings this past month?

PERSONAL REFLECTION ON ANY MOVEMENT EXPERIENCED IN STRESS REDUCTION

- In moving from high stress to moderate stress (5—>3)?

- In moving from moderate stress to joy (3—>1)?

- In expanding the joy I was already experiencing (1—>1)?

Appendix B:
How to Deal with Stress:
33 Tips That Work

(Source: Henrik Edberg, How to Deal with Stress: 33 Tips That Work, http://www.positivityblog.com/how-to-deal-with-stress/)

Henrik Edberg shares some constructive habits for dealing with stressful situations as they arise. He cites 33 behaviors that have become habits for him and have been an important aid for living a less stressful life.

1. One thing at a time.

2. Write everything down.

3. Keep your daily to-do list very short.

4. Don't make mountains out of molehills.

5. Spend 80% of your time focusing on a solution.

6. Ask instead of guessing.

7. Pack your bag before you go to sleep.

8. Balance fully focused work with complete rest.

9. Set clear boundaries for your day.

10. Disconnect over the weekend.

11. Make sure you take time to do what you love to do.

12. Delegate.

13. Eliminate.

14. Be 10 minutes early.

15. Stay on track by asking yourself questions every day.

16. Let your lunch be a slow time of relaxing.

17. Keep a very simple workspace.

18. Build a zone of few distractions for your work hours.

19. Get done with something that stresses or bothers you.

20. If it does not get done, then there is a day tomorrow too.

21. Everything in its place.

22. Check your email etc. just once and as late in the workday as possible.

23. Limit your daily information intake.

24. Listen to yourself.

25. Be here in the present moment.

26. Stop trying to do things perfectly.

27. Ask for help.

28. Talk it out with someone.

29. Zoom out by asking, "Is there anyone on the planet having it worse than me right now?"

30. Slow down.

31. Tell yourself: "Just take care of today."

32. Just breathe.

33. Be smart about the three fundamentals of energy: sleeping, eating, and exercising.

Appendix C:
25 Classical Musical Works
on Joy

The following are offered as some of the best classical pieces of music that, in my opinion, relate beautifully to the expression of joy.

1. Symphony No. 9 in D Minor, Op. 125, "Choral":
    Ode and der Freude (Ode to Joy)

2. The Four Seasons (Le Quattro Stagioni), Op. 8 -
    Concerto No. 1 for Violin and Strings in E Major, RV 269,
    "Spring": I. Allegro

3. Music for the Royal Fireworks, HWV 351: III.
    La réjouissance

4. Chorale from Cantata BWV 147: Jesu bleibet meine
    Freude (Jesu, Joy of Man's Desiring)

5. An der Schönen Blauen Donau (On the Beautiful Blue
    Danube), Op. 314: Waltz (excerpt)

6. Symphony No. 94 in G Major, Hob. I:94, "Surprise":
    II. Andante

7. Serenade No. 13 in G Major, K. 525, "Eine Kleine
    Nachtmusik": IV. Rondo: Allegro

8. Wilhelm Tell (William Tell): Overture (excerpt)

9. Le Nozze di Figaro (The Marriage of Figaro),
    K. 492: Overture

10. A Midsummer Night's Dream, Op. 61: IX.
    Wedding March

11. The Messiah, HWV 56: Hallelujah Chorus

12. Brandenburg Concerto No. 3 in G Major, BWV 1048:
    I. Allegro

13. String Quintet No. 5 in E Major, Op. 11: III. Minuet

14. Orphée aux enfers (Orpheus in the Underworld):
    Can-can

15. Sylvia Suite: Pizzicato

16. Solomon, HWV 67: The Arrival of the Queen of Sheba

17. Pomp and Circumstance, Five Marches for Orchestra,
    Op. 39: No. 1 in D Major, "Land of Hope and Glory"

18. Water Music Suite No. 2 in D Major, HWV 349:
    II. Alla Hornpipe

19. Coppélia: Festive Dance and Waltz of the Hours

20. Partita No. 3 in E Major for Solo Violin, BWV 1006:
    I. Preludio

21. The Planets, Suite for Large Orchestra, Op. 32: Jupiter,
    The Bringer of Jollity

22. Carmen Suite No. 1: Les Toreadors

23. Suite de Symphonies No. 1: Fanfare-Rondeau

24. Radetzky-March, Op. 228

25. Festival Overture in E-Flat Major, "The Year 1812",
    Op. 49

Appendix D: 25 Poems on Joy

The following are offered as some of the best poetry that, in my opinion, relate beautifully to the expression of joy.

1. "Walt Whitman" by Walt Whitman
2. "The Growth of Love" by Robert Seymour
3. "Love" by William Wordsworth
4. "Song of the Open Road" by Walt Whitman
5. "The Marriage of Heaven and Hell" by William Blake
6. "The Dream" by George (Lord) Byron
7. "The Triumph of Life" by Percy Bysshe Shelley
8. "Hyperion" by John Keats
9. "The Idiot Boy" by William Wordsworth
10. "Howl" by Allen Ginsberg
11. "Humanitad" by Oscar Wilde
12. "The Ballad of the White Horse" by G.K. Chesterton
13. "Poem of Joys" Walt Whitman
14. "The Hunting of the Snark" by Lewis Carroll
15. "White Flock" by Anna Akhmatova
16. "The Knights Tale" by Geoffrey Chaucer
17. "Lara" by George (Lord) Byron
18. "Inferno" (English) by Dante Alighieri
19. "The Most Beautiful Woman In Town" by Charles Bukowski
20. "Ravenna" by Oscar Wilde
21. "The Walk" by Friedrich von Schiller
22. "The Dungeon" by William Wordsworth
23. "The Seasons: Winter" by James Thomson
24. "The Holy Grail" by Alfred Lord Tennyson
25. "The White Cliffs" by Alice Duer Miller

Appendix E:
10 Paintings on Joy

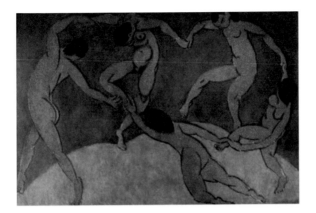

Henri Matisse, *Dance II*, 1910.

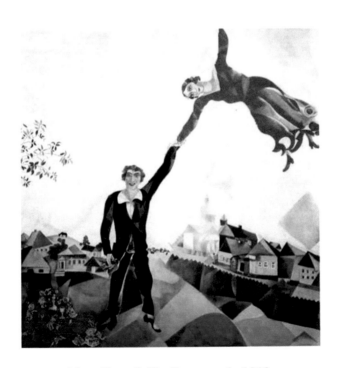

Marc Chagall, *The Promenade*, 1918.

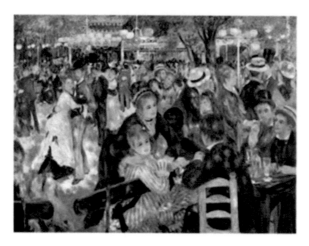

Pierre Auguste Renoir, *Bal du moulin de la Galette,* 1876.

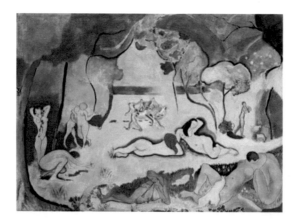

Henri Matisse, *Le bonheur de vivre, (The Joy of Life),* 1905.

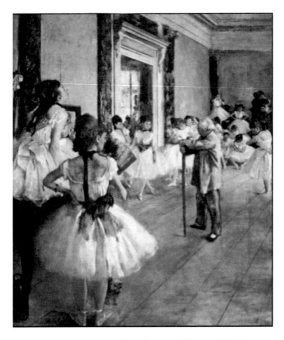

Edgar Degas, *The Dance Class*, 1874.

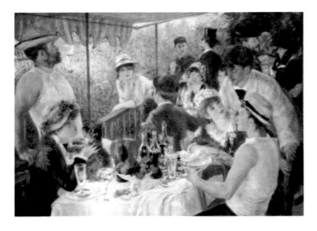

Pierre Auguste Renoir, *Luncheon of the Boating Party*, 1875.

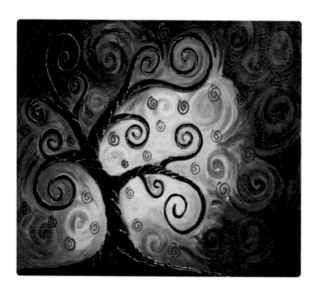

Michelle D'Oyley, *Twisted with Joy,* n.d.

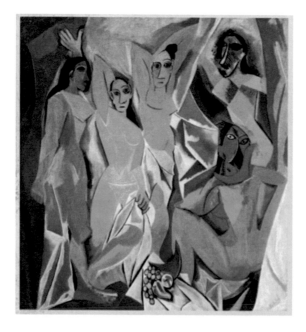

Picasso, *Les Demoiselles d'Avignon,* 1907.

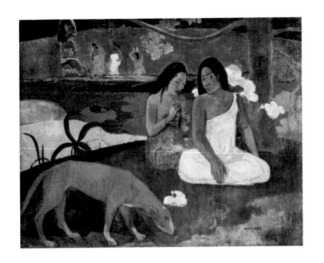

Paul Gauguin, *Arearea*, 1892.

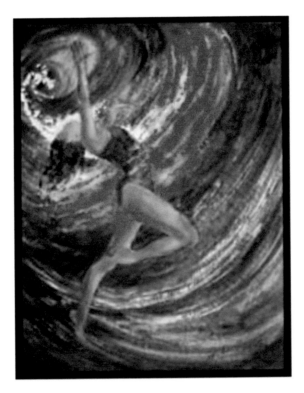

Joy Ann Cabanos, *Ascendo*, n.d.

Appendix F:
Concerning Contemplation

THREE WAYS TO ACCESS THE SILENCE

It was Teresa Ávila who spoke of three types of prayer and each involving the brain in different ways. It is contemplative prayer and the quieting of the mind so it can rest in awareness in the present that characterizes the most profound presence to the divine.

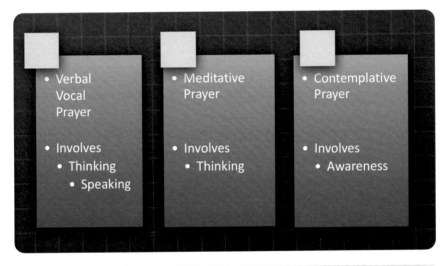

- Verbal Vocal Prayer

- Involves
  - Thinking
    - Speaking

- Meditative Prayer

- Involves
  - Thinking

- Contemplative Prayer

- Involves
  - Awareness

CHOOSING A SACRED WORD

The sacred word is a symbol both of your intention to be with God in the silence and to live out of the presence that was experienced. Thus, if your experience was one of calm and tranquility, you could carry that state of being into the actions of your day. If it were love and support you experienced, that would then be what is brought forth in actions of the day. It should be mentioned that in the act of living out the energy or grace of the presence, you have become an instrument of that grace in God's hands, and you are creating that same presence in others. Expect great outcomes from such impactful prayer!

TOOLS, OBSTACLES, AND STEPS

Think of it as an exercise in addition: 2+2=4. Thus, 2 tools of a sacred word or mantra + breathing in and out deeply = your disposing yourself to God's presence. While in that state of presence or awareness, 2 obstacles will arise that keep you from remaining there. They are distractions or thinking about other things. The more you are able to let distractions and thoughts float by your consciousness, as a canoe down a river, the more you'll be able to remain in awareness and in the presence. The 4 steps then are: having a mantra or sacred word, breathing deeply to relaxation, synchronizing the word to the breathing, letting go and floating into the presence.

> **2 Tools**
> **+ 2 Obstacles**
> _____
> **4 Steps**
>
> **2 Tools = (1) Mantra + (2) Breathing**
> **2 Obstacles = (1) Distraction or (2) Thinking**
> **4 Steps = (1) Mantra (2) Sync (3) Ascent (4) Float**

GOING INTO THE PRESENCE

It is the tools of Sacred Word and Breathing that dispose you to saying "yes" to God and entering the silence as an "Ascent." The "work" of the individual is to dispose oneself to God's presence. God will do the rest, for God is always present and available as unconditional love. It is we who are not disposed to that presence.

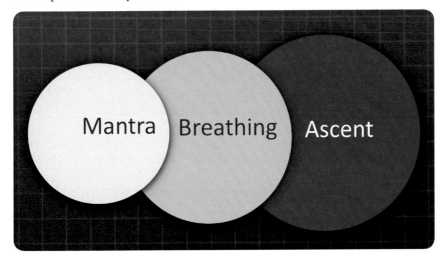

OVERCOMING DISTRACTIONS AND THINKING

The two obstacles that keep us from being present in awareness are distractions and thinking. Both take us out of any possible unitive experience. Think of gazing at a stunning sunset and the awe of just being one with it. That is a unitive experience. The minute you begin thinking about it or calling someone to view it with you, you become the-subject-thinking, and the sunset has become the object. You are no longer with it. The unitive experience has been broken. Non-intrusive distractions like an air handler or light traffic outside can be let go of easily. However, a crying baby or construction noise is much more of a challenge. With compulsive thinking, try becoming the witness to your thinking, as in, "Look at silly me! I just can't let that go. Now settle down. There'll be lots of time to think that through later." Another way to handle compulsive thinking is simply to concentrate on your breathing. You can't think of two things at the same time. The tools will be used each time you are distracted or begin thinking and may have to be used many times during a single sitting.

- **Integration of Mild Distractions, e.g. traffic, HVAC, birds, rain, etc.**

- **Kinds of Thinking**
  - **Remembering to Do Something**
  - **Planning**
  - **Worry**
  - **Day Dreaming**

- **Compulsive Thinking**
  - **The Witness**
  - **Think about Your Breathing**

SITTING IN SILENCE

To have a contemplative practice is to acquire a daily habit of sitting in silence (S-I-S) using the two tools and the four steps mentioned in this appendix. Deep breathing is itself a teacher for you to know what to do, for as you breathe deeply, your abdomen comes in, your shoulders go back, and your chin goes up a bit. These three actions allow for a clear path of air and full expansion of the lungs. To completely relax on your exhale, simply relax your forehead, soften your eyes, and unclench your jaw. Repeat this process until completely relaxed. Breathing never felt so good!

- 4 Steps = (1) Mantra (2) Sync (3) Ascent (4) Float

- Breathing In (Intuitively Self-Taught)
  - Abdomen →In
  - Shoulders →Back
  - Chin → Up

- Breathing Out (Intuitively Self-Taught)
  - Forehead → Relax
  - Eyes →Soften
  - Jaw → Release

COMING OUT OF THE SILENCE

After a sitting of 10, 20, or 30 minutes, it is time to come out of the presence. A chime on a timer is a helpful thing to have. It will keep you from having to think about how much time has passed or how much remains. Once you are back to your awareness in the room, describe the experience of the presence to yourself. Was it calm, warm, affirming, luminous, etc.? From the experience, create an intention of how your experience of the presence might be made into an intention for the day. Thus, if I felt affirmed and loved, how or to whom might I affirm to show love in a special way today? If it was warmth and acceptance, who might I determine to be the recipient of that same warmth and acceptance? In this way, you experience prayer that makes a difference, and contemplative prayer has become contemplative action.

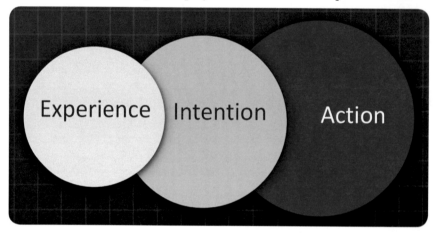

Appendix G: 5 Breathing Exercises to Lower Your Stress Levels

(Source: https://adrenalfatiguesolution.com/5-simple-breathing-exercises/)

It is medical research and our own physiological experience that attest to the fact that breathing deeply can actually lower our level of stress at any given moment. There is simple relief for the myriads of folks who experience stress every day. If we are to remain healthy, deep breathing is a good part of the answer for the relief of stress. The following are five simple breathing exercises to help us do that, and they can be done almost anywhere and at any time stress is being experienced.

BELLY BREATHING

The first thing you need to learn to do is what's called Belly Breathing. This is the most basic of the breathing methods we have at our disposal, and, therefore, is the one you should master before trying out the others. It's very simple and requires just a few steps:

1. Sit down comfortably or lie down on a yoga mat, depending on your personal preference.

2. Place one of your hands on your stomach, just below your ribcage. Place the second hand over your chest.

3. Breathe in deeply through your nostrils, letting your first hand be pushed out by your stomach. You should find that your chest stays stationary.

4. Breathe out through your lips, pursing them as if you were about to whistle. Gently guide the hand on your stomach inwards, helping to press out the breath.

5. Slowly repeat between three and 10 times.

You should begin to feel relaxed as soon as you have repeated the Belly Breathing exercise two or three times, but keep going for as long as you feel you need. After you have mastered this breathing exercise, there are four additional methods for you to try, ranging in difficulty.

4-7-8 BREATHING

The method that we call 4-7-8 Breathing also requires you to be sitting down or lying comfortably. Here are the steps you need to follow:

1. Get into the same position as you did for the Belly Breathing exercise, with one hand on your stomach and one on your chest.

2. Breathe in slowly but deeply. Take four seconds to breathe in, feeling your stomach move in the process.

3. Hold your breath for seven seconds.

4. Breathe out as silently as you can manage, taking eight seconds. Once you reach eight, you should have emptied your lungs of air.

Repeat as many times as you need, making sure to stick to the 4-7-8 pattern.

ROLL BREATHING

If you are looking for a breathing exercise which you can do comfortably sitting down, try the Roll Breathing method. Its aim is not just to relax, but also to encourage the full use of your lung capacity. Beginners are advised to lie down, but after your first time, you should find it just as easy to sit and complete this exercise. Follow these steps:

1. Position yourself with your left hand on your stomach, and place your right hand over your chest. Your hands should move as you inhale and exhale.

2. Take a deep breath from your lower lungs; breathe slowly ensuring that the hand over your chest doesn't move as you take the breath. Make sure you are using your nose to breathe in, and then exhale using your mouth.

3. Repeat the deep breath up to eight times. On the ninth repetition, once you have filled your lower lungs, take a breath, which will move your chest up, as you would normally breathe. This will fill your entire lung capacity.

4. Gently exhale through your mouth, being sure to empty your lungs as you do so. While you exhale, make a small whooshing noise. You should notice that both of your hands are moving back towards your body as your stomach and chest fall.

5. You should practice this method for between four and five minutes. When you exhale, you should be able to feel a tangible difference in your stress levels.

MORNING BREATHING

While the above three exercises can be completed whenever necessary, the next method is called Morning Breathing, and as the name suggests, should be practiced once you have woken up. It aims to relax your muscles after a good night's sleep and will help you to minimize tension for the remainder of the day – so you can start as you mean to go on.

Here are the steps to follow:

1. Stand up straight, and slightly bending your knees, bend your torso forward from the waist. Your arms should be hanging close to the floor, limply.

2. Take a breath in slowly, returning to your original standing position. You should look like an inflatable ghost you may see at Halloween: your head should be the last thing to straighten up.

3. Exhale, returning to the position of being bent forward by the end of your exhale. Stand up straight once you have finished, stretching your muscles as required.

DEEP MUSCLE RELAXATION & BELLY BREATHING

Finally, the Deep Muscle Relaxation technique is the most time-consuming but can also be the most rewarding for your body. This works best when combined with the Belly Breathing that I mentioned earlier and is a great way to attain the *relaxation response*. You will exercise each major muscle in turn, but pay most attention to any muscles that are causing discomfort or ache.

To start, sit down in a comfortable position and focus on your Belly Breathing, closing your eyes, if need be. Then do the following:

- To relax your face, knit your eyebrows together and release.

- To relax your neck tilt your head down towards your neck, and push your chin to your chest, then release.

- To relax your shoulders, make a shrugging motion, then release.

- To relax your arms, push both arms away from your torso, stretch them out and then relax them by your side.

- To relax your legs, point your toes as far away as they will stretch and then relax.

All of these stretches should be conducted at the same time as the Belly Breathing we covered earlier. Breathe long and deep, and take your time with each stretch.

Appendix H:
The State of Being Awake

(Source: Richard Rohr's Daily Meditation for Thursday, February 9, 2017)

When we are able to simply sit in silence, the state we acquire is closer to wakefulness than it is to sleep. This is the clarion call of Eastern and Western mystics, or in common parlance, to "Wake up and smell the roses." Contemporary writers in spirituality, such as Rohr, Keating, Bourgeault, and Tolle, offer "how to's" for achieving this waking up.

They include:

- Separation of the self that is me from the mental activity going on in my head to become the observer or witness of my own thoughts

- To notice or pay attention to thoughts in my mind, as if they were boats passing by on a river

- To be a calm observer of my behavior, as if I were watching a video of myself in the past

- To give the child within me a voice so he/she might speak to the adult within, and the latter could look upon the child with heartfelt compassion and understanding

- To surrender, sink, or free fall, into pure awareness with no particular object in mind. This is akin to Jesus' invitation to, **"Lose oneself in order to find oneself."** (Luke 9:24)

The impact of such awakening is a larger, fuller sense of who I am, and it is as if my skin becomes porous, and I assume a greater sense of self. It feels good, true, and beautiful. This self has a feeling of "groundedness." I am as nothing and yet as everything. One, joined with all of creation. This larger sense of self is what religious traditions call the soul, the true self, or the collective unconscious. Mystics have learned that it is not I who am doing anything here, but what is happening in awareness is somehow being done to me and by a force beyond me. In the process, I become the vessel, and the energy that is experienced flows through me to others via my awareness, intentions, and actions. In this, the mind of Jesus Christ and my mind are one, and scripture comes to pass: "Let this mind be in you, which was also in Christ Jesus. In your relationships with one another, have the same mindset **as Christ Jesus.**" (Philippians 2:5)

Appendix I:
45 Fruits and Flowers
of the Presence Practice

(Source: Michael Brown, The Presence Process: A journey into present moment awareness, (Vancouver, Canada), 2010, 244–72.)

Michael Brown lists 45 "fruits and flowers" that are a result of what he calls "the Presence Process." He states,

> "The Presence Process is a guided journey that provides the practical techniques and perceptual tools required to extract our attention from the trappings of a time-based mentality, allowing us to gradually re-enter the present moment in which our experience is unfolding." (p. xxiii)

1. We respond instead of reacting
2. We have more energy
3. We overcome procrastination
4. We complete tasks efficiently, effortlessly, and feel as though we have more time in which to accomplish them
5. We no longer hurry
6. Working conditions become more enjoyable
7. We are less resistant to the unpredictable currents of life
8. We experience spontaneous creativity
9. We feel more comfortable around our immediate family
10. Circumstances and people that once annoyed us no longer take up our attention
11. Our intimate relationships improve
12. We stop interfering in other people's lives
13. Our sleep is more restful
14. Nagging symptoms we may have experienced for years are integrated
15. Longtime habits cease
16. We lose weight without dieting
17. We enjoy being around children
18. We laugh more and are more playful

19. Our diet gravitates effortlessly toward eating healthily
20. We take active interest in our health
21. People are attracted to us and enjoy our company
22. We enjoy solitude
23. We sense events before they occur
24. We experience synchronicity in the events of life
25. We experience greater abundance
26. We feel less inclined to plan the future
27. We spring-clean our house and let go of "stuff" we have hoarded for years
28. We manifest less drama
29. Certain people move out of our sphere of activity
30. Our outlook is naturally optimistic
31. We become interested in our vibrational well-being
32. We cease seeking distraction
33. We are more gentle and compassionate toward ourselves
34. We experience less anxiety
35. We are more compassionate and have more patience with others
36. Our life becomes a journey and not an intended destination
37. We experience spontaneous gratitude
38. What we require comes to us instead of our seeking it out
39. We feel a deeper sense of connection with nature
40. We become part of the natural cycles
41. We perceive the window dressing of the world
42. We no longer seek the extraordinary
43. Our capacity for trusting our insight blossoms
44. We feel blessed with purpose
45. We make an authentic contribution to this world

Appendix J:
Concerning Planning

The following questions could serve as both a baseline after reading this book, as well as a check on your progress over time.

1. What are your greatest sources of stress in these days?

_____

_____

_____

_____

2. What are your most effective means of dealing with them at this particular time?

_____

_____

_____

_____

3. What are your present prayer practices?

_____

_____

_____

_____

4. How can they be improved?

_____

_____

_____

_____

5. What can you say about the following equation as it relates to your life today? Stress management + prayer practice —> reclaiming joy within

_____

_____

_____

_____

6. What would be the elements of a plan for reclaiming more joy in your life in moving forward today?

_____

_____

_____

_____

How to use this appendix:

- *As a weekly review within a Holy Hour*
- *As a reflection piece for a Monthly Day-in-the-Desert or a meeting with your Spiritual Director*
- *As an annual review while on a retreat*

Appendix K:
The Ignatian Examen
as a Stress Reliever

(Source: Through All the Days of Life by Nick Schiro, S.J.)

Practice: This is my take on Ignatius' original examen and further refined by Nick Schiro. It divides the daily examen into two parts. One part — before the bold line below — in the morning, and the second part — after the bold line — in the evening. I believe that it allows for a greater intentionality for the day and a more thorough reflection on what has happened in the course of the day.

	Gratitude (Morning)	Petition (Morning)	Review (Evening)	Forgiveness (Evening)	Renewal (Evening)
	• *All's a gift* • **For what am I most grateful?**	• *Help me be more honest* • **What do I really want?**	• *What's happening to me today?* • **How've I experienced God's love today?**	• *I'm still learning to grow in love* • **What have been my inadequate choices today?**	• *Help me look with longing to the future* • **How might today lead to a brighter tomorrow?**
Monday Date					
Tuesday Date					
Wednesday Date					
Thursday Date					
Friday Date					
Saturday Date					
Sunday Date					

Appendix L: Invitation to Join an Online Weekly Contemplative Prayer Group

CENTERING PRAYER

- Opens us to the divine presence
- Gives us a powerful resource to live out of that presence
- Creates transformation in ourselves and our relationships with others

OUR PURPOSE AS A WEEKLY CONTEMPLATIVE PRAYER COMMUNITY

- To deepen our commitment to Centering Prayer
- To have our weekly practice become a habitual practice for our own personal prayer
- To have a community of weekly support in the half-hour we pray together
- To connect via (1) text messages and (2) the *Insight Timer* app for smartphones

As a prayer community, we interact via text messages, so we invite you to join our group via your cell phone number. Any of the three of us is very happy to add you to our text message group. While we have set up our group called "Living in the Presence of Christ" as a group on the *Insight Timer* app, you do not have to be part of the *Insight Timer* group, although that could be helpful to you. If you do choose to be part of *Insight Timer*, you can post comments there regarding how the session went. Over time, you will have a written record of our growth together as an online community of contemplative prayer.

All that said, the simplest way to join is to email or text one of us your interest, name, and cell phone number, and we will guide you one-on-one regarding next steps.

This Invitation

- Is for busy folks who want to pray contemplatively with others once a week

- Involves little or no preparation

- Allows you to spend 30 minutes of silence with a group of other Christians each week

- Meets every Tuesday morning, 6:00–6:30 am (Eastern Standard Time)

- Apart from using text messages as a connection, we also use the *Insight Timer* app as a vehicle that further unites us in God's presence, offering us a written text history of our weekly interactions

- Is "guilt free": Not every person will be able to participate every week; if you need to miss a week due to a schedule change, simply join when you can. However, the more consistent you are in your personal prayer life, the more you will benefit.

HOW IT WORKS:

- An individual has a desire to experience God's presence regularly

- The person wants to live out of the experience of that graced presence

- There is an openness to surface a Sacred Word before we begin the weekly silence together

- The individual receives a bit more of instruction in Centering Prayer each week we pray

- We follow the teachings of Fr. Thomas Keating, C.O.S.O. on www.contemplativeoutreach.org

2 STEPS ON "HOW TO GET CONNECTED"

1. Email one of the following Team Leaders, and they will connect you to our special text message group, as well as introduce you to the *Insight Timer* app, if you are unfamiliar with it.

   Nicholas Amato: FatherNicholasAmato@gmail.com

   Pringle Franklin: franklin.pringle@comcast.net

   Dr. Ann Kulze: ann@drannwellness.com

2. The following are the instructions for using the *Insight Timer* App on your smartphone:

   - Download the app as you do any of your other apps.
   - Open to the *Insight Timer* homepage.
   - Click on the icon of 4 dots at the bottom of the screen. It represents "groups."
   - Because one of our team leaders added you to our *Insight Timer* group, you will then be able to see our group "Living in Christ's Presence."
   - Click on it.
   - In the upper right hand corner of the screen is a black oval with the word "Post" and a pencil in it.
   - Click on it and tell us you've made it to the portal of our group.
   - We can then welcome you to the group, thus notifying others that you are now part of our contemplative prayer community.

COMMITMENT

- To join us on Tuesday 6:00–6:30 a.m., as you are able.

- To commit to doing this for a three-month period (Beginning or renewable any Jan. 1st, Apr. 1st, Jul. 1st, or Oct. 1st). We're not "enforcers"; this is just a suggestion to support you in your desire to commit to a regular practice of contemplative prayer.

- Each week you are cordially invited to think of a sacred word and, if you care to, to ask the group to pray for an intention. This can be done using a text message or posting on the *Insight Timer* app.

- There are absolutely no fees or obligations. This is just a group of Christians who want to deepen their desire to pray together contemplatively.

- There is an invitation after our half-hour of contemplative presence to make a private intention regarding an action you will take that day to live out the experience of God's presence you have just had.

AFTER 3 MONTHS

- You can take a break from the group.

- Try it on your own.

- Or just unsubscribe for no stated reason.

- You may "reconnect" for any three-month period (beginning every Jan. 1st, Apr. 1st, Jul. 1st, or Oct. 1st) when the Spirit moves you.

Bibliography

"2015 Stress in America," *American Psychological Association*, accessed, December 5, 2016, http://www.apa.org/news/press/releases/ stress/2015/snapshot.aspx.

Deanne Alban, "12 Effects of Chronic Stress on Your Brain," *Be Brain Fit,* accessed December 7, 2016, https://bebrainfit.com/effects-chronic-stress-brain/.

Nicholas Amato, *Living in God: Contemplative Prayer and Contemplative Action,* (Bloomington: WestBow Press, 2016).

Jordan Aumann, O.P. "St. Teresa's Teaching on the Grades of Prayer," *Catholic Culture,* accessed January 18, 2017, www.catholicculture.org/ culture/library/view.cfm?id=7725.

Gillian Bethel, *From Stress to Joy,* (Roseville: Amazing Facts, Inc., 2004), 317.

Bible: New American Bible (Revised Edition).

Bible: New American Standard Bible.

Bible: New International Version.

Cynthia Bourgeault, "The Beatitudes, Be Peaceable, Be Free," April 21, 2017, *Center for Action and Contemplation,* accessed April 29, 2017, https://cac.org/be-peaceable-be-free-2017-04-21/.

———, *The Holy Trinity and the Law of Three,* (Boston: Shambhala, 2013).

———, *The Shape of God: Deepening the Mystery of the Trinity* (Center for Action and Contemplation: 2005), disc 4 (CD, DVD, MP3 download).

———, *The Wisdom Jesus: Transforming Heart and Mind—A New Perspective on Christ and His Message,* (Boston: Shambhala, 2008).

Richard Brittain, "Vaughan Williams' The Lark Ascending", *YouTube,* accessed April 6, 2017, https://www.youtube.com/watch?v=ZR2JlDnT2l8.

Michael Brown, *The Presence Process* (Vancouver: Namaste Publishing, 2005).

Joseph Campbell, *The Power of Myth,* (New York: Anchor Publishing, 1991).

The Catechism of the Catholic Church.

"Marc Chagall," *Yahoo Answers,* accessed April 7, 2017, https://answers. yahoo.com/question/index?qid=20100203082601AACbpVi.

The Cloud of Unknowing, introductory commentary and translation by Ira Progoff translated by Ira Progroff, (New York: Delta Books, 1957).

Unknown Mystic, *The Cloud of Unknowing,* (New Kensington: Whitaker House, 2014).

"The Cortical Lottery: Dopamine and the Activity Set-Point," *Myosynthesis,* last modified March 3, 2011, accessed December 10, 2016, www. myosynthesis.com/cortical-lottery-dopamine-activity-setpoint.

Marshall Craver, Faculty Member of the Shalem Institute, Washington, D.C., phone conversation, February 9, 2017.

The Dalai Lama. An Open Heart: Practicing Compassion in Everyday Life, (Little, Brown and Co., 2001), 91.

Antonio Damasio, "The Quest to Understand Consciousness," *TED Talk,* March 2011, accessed April 18, 2017, https://www.ted.com/talks/ antonio_damasio_the_quest_to_ understand consciousness.

Lucien Deiss, CSSp, "Grant to Us O Lord," *YouTube,* February 22, 2015, accessed April 25, 2017, https://www.youtube.com/ watch?v=PxkTLzgNZsw.

Mitch Ditkoff, "50 Awesome Quotes on Risk Taking," *Huffington Post,* accessed April 21, 2017, last updated November 10, 2016, http:// www.huffingtonpost.com/mitch-ditkoff/50-awesome-quotes-on-risk_b_2078573.html.

Charles Duhigg, *The Power of Habit: Why We Do What We Do in Life and Business,"* (New York: Random House Trade Paperbacks, 2012).

T.S. Eliot, *"East Coker,"* accessed February 5, 2017, http://www.coldbacon. com/poems/fq.html.

"Examples of Reasoning," *Reference,* accessed January 30, 2017, www. reference.com.

James Finley, *Christian Meditation: Experiencing the Presence of God* (New York: HarperSanFrancisco, 2004).

———, Exclusive Center for Action and Contemplation Living School curriculum, Unit 1.

———, "Transforming Trauma: Exploring the Spiritual Dimensions of Healing," Manuscript. Gerry May Shalem Seminar. April 24-25, 2015.

"The Four Brain States," *Tools for Wellness,* accessed December 7, 2016, http://www.toolsforwellness.com/brainstates.html.

"The Four Truths," *PBS*, http://www.pbs.org/edens/thailand/buddhism.htm.

Pope Francis, "Handling Stress," *The Guardian*, accessed April 29, 2017, https://www.theguardian.com/world/2017/feb/09/pope-francis-reveals-how-he-shrugs-off-stress-im-not-on-tranquilisers.

———, "Homily of Pope Francis," *Vatican*, accessed March 15, 2017, http://w2.vatican.va/content/francesco/en/homilies/2013/documents/papa-francesco_20130324_palme.html.

Mandy Mayfield, "Meeting with Donald Trump," *Washington Examiner*, http://www.washingtonexaminer.com/pope-on-meeting-with-trump-i-never-make-a-judgement-about-a-person-without-hearing-him-out/article/2623043.

Reginald Garrigou-Lagrange, "The Three Ages of the Spiritual Life According to the Fathers and the Great Spiritual Writers," *The Three Ages of the Interior Life*, accessed January 28, 2017, http://www.christianperfection.info/tta26.php.

Andrew Harvey and Carolyn Baker, *Return to Joy,* (Bloomington: iUniverse, Bloomington, 2016).

The author is unknown. The English Augustinian mystic Walter Hilton has been suggested. Some claim the author was a Carthusian priest.

"The Holmes and Rahe Stress Scale: Understanding the Impact of Long Term Stress," *MindTool,* accessed December 7, 2016, https://www.mindtools.com/pages/article/newTCS_82.htm.

Gerard Manley Hopkins, "The Golden Echo," *Bartleby*, accessed April 5, 2017, http://www.bartleby.com/122/36.html.

———, "Morning Midday and Evening Sacrifice," *Famous Poets and Poems*, access April 5, 2017, http://www.famouspoetsandpoems.com/poets/gerard_manley_hopkins/poems/13995.

https://www.catholicculture.org/culture/library/view.cfm?id=7725.

http://www.psychologyofjoy.com.

https://www.themystica.com, (December 5, 2016).

Todd Kashdan and Robert Biswas-Diener, "Join the grouchy club: Why negative emotions can be a force for good," *Mail Online*, last modified January 3, 2015, accessed March 15, 2017, http://www. dailymail.co.uk/home/you/article-2894291/Join-grouchy-club-negative-emotions-force-good.html.

Thomas Keating, *Open Mind, Open Heart. Continuum: The Contemplative Dimension of the Gospel*, (New York: Continuum International Publishing Group, 2006), 58.

———, *Reflections on the Unknowable*, (Brooklyn: Lantern Books, 2014).

Peter Kreeft, accessed December 5, 2016, http://www.peterkreeft.com/ topics/joy.htm.

C. S. Lewis, *Surprised by Joy: The Shape of My Early Life.* (Orlando: Harcourt, 1955).

"The link between stress and forgetfulness," *Women's Health Network*, accessed December 7, 2016, http://www.womenshealthnetwork. com/adrenal-fatigue-and-stress/the-link-between-stress-and-forgetfulness.aspx

Merriam Webster Dictionary, s.v. accessed December 5, 2016, http://www. merriam-webster.com.

Liturgy of the Hours **CITATION**

Ignatius of Loyola, "The examen."

Catherine Mowry LaCugna, *God for Us: The Trinity and Christian Life,* (New York: HarperSanFrancisco, 1991).

Andrew Louth, *Modern Orthodox Thinkers: From the Philokalia to the Present,* (Downers Grove: Intervarsity Press, 2015), 1. For a complete text of the Philokalia see: *The Philokalia, Volume 4: The Complete Text; Compiled by St. Nikodimos of the Holy Mountain & St. Markarios of Corinth* translated by G.E.H. Palmer, Sherrard, Kallistos and Ware, (London: Faber and Faber, 1999).

Jim Marion, *Putting on the Mind of Christ: The Inner Work of Christian Spirituality* (Charlottesville: Hampton Roads Publishing Company, 2000.

Louis Marko, *The Life and Writings of C. S. Lewis (The Great Courses)*, CD, (The Teaching Company, 2000).

James Martin, S.J., *The Jesuit Guide to (Almost) Everything: A Spirituality for Real Life,* (San Francisco: HarperOne, 2012).

Henri Matisse, *The Joy of Life, Wikiart*, accessed April 17, 2017, https://www.wikiart.org/en/henri-matisse/the-joy-of-life-1906.

Laurel Mellin, *Wired for Joy: A Revolutionary Method for Creating Happiness from Within,* (Hays House, 2010).

John Main, "Everything you need to know about how to meditate in 128 words:," accessed January 21, 2017, www.johnmain.org.

Mepkin Priest Wellness Program is a week of intensive training in prayer, nutrition, exercise and community for Catholic priests and began at Mepkin Trappist Abbey in South Carolina.

Merriam Webster Dictionary, s.v., http://www.merriam-webster.com.

"Mystic," *Online Google Dictionary*, accessed February 3, 2017, http://google-dictionary.so8848.com.

Razali Salleh Mohd, "Life Event, Stress and Illness," *The Malaysian Journal of Medical Sciences,* accessed December 7, 2016, https://www.ncbi.nlm.nih.gov/pmc/articles/PMC3341916/.

Julian of Norwich, "Julian of Norwich Quotes," *AZ Quotes*, accessed January 15, 2017, http://www.azquotes.com/author/17697-Julian_of_Norwich.

"Nuptial Blessing from the Catholic Marriage Ritual," *For Your Marriage*, accessed January 28, 2017, http://www.foryourmarriage.org/the-nuptial-blessing/.

"Our Beliefs," *Center for Spiritual Living*, accessed February 3, 2017, http://www.cslftlauderdale.org/our-beliefs/.

Raimon Panikkar, *Christophany: Fullness of Man,* (New York: Orbis Books, 2004).

Pablo Picasso, *Guernica,* 1937.

Narjis Pierre, "When Compassion Fills My Heart," *Compassionate San Antonio*, accessed April 20, 2017, http://sacompassionnet.org/poem-when-compassion-fills-my-heart/.

Theodore Roethke, "The Rose," *The Collected Poems of Theodore Roethke,* (New York: Anchor Books, 1974).

Maria Popova, "Wendell Berry on Solitude and Why Pride and Despair Are Two Great Enemies of Creative Work," *Two-Handed Warriors*, January 4, 2015, accessed April 25, 2017, http://garydavidstratton. com/2015/01/04/wendell-berry-on-solitude-and-why-pride-and-despair-are-the-two-great-enemies-of-creative-work/.

———, "A Benediction on the World: Wendall Barry on Creaturely Joy," *Brainpickings*, https://www.brainpickings.org/2016/08/02/ wendell-berry-great-blue-heron/.

Bible: Revised Standard Version.

Richard of St. Victor, *The Book of the Patriarchs, The Mystical Ark, Book Three of the Trinity* (Classics of Western Spirituality), (Mahwah: Paulist Press, 1979), 387-389.

Richard Rohr, "Being Human," Richard Rohr's Daily Meditation, , February 21, 2017, accessed April 20, 2017, https://cac.org/ being-human-2017-02-21/. Adapted from James Finley, *Christian Meditation: Experiencing the Presence of God,* (New York: 2004).

———, *Everything Belongs: The Gift of Contemplative Prayer* (New York: The Crossroad Publishing Company, 1999).

———, "Experience: Weekly Summary," *Richard Rohr's Daily Meditation*, January 28, 2017, accessed January 28, 2017, https://cac.org/ experience-weekly-summary-2017-01-28/.

———, "Knowing through Loving," Richard Rohr's Daily Mediation, February 16, 2017, accessed April 17, 2017, https://cac.org/knowing-through-loving-2017-02-26/.

———, "Perennial Wisdom," *Richard Rohr's Daily Meditation*, January 15, 2017, accessed January 15, 2017, https://cac.org/experience-weekly-summary-2017-01-28/.

———, "Spirituality of Imperfection: Week 2 Summary: Sunday, July 24-Friday, July 29, 2016," *Richard Rohr's Daily Meditation*, July 30, 2016, accessed January 19, 2017, https://cac.org/spirituality-imperfection-week-2-summary-2016-07-30/.

———, "The Third Way," Richard Rohr's Daily Meditation", August 26, 2016, accessed January 31, 2017, https://cac.org/the-third-way-2016-08-26/.

Adapted from Richard Rohr, *Yes, And…: Daily Meditations* (Cincinatti: Franciscan Media, 2013).

Richard Rohr with Mike Morrell, *The Divine Dance: The Trinity and Your Transformation,* (New Kensington: Whitaker House, 2016).

Jerry Rosser, "Psychology of Joy," accessed December 5, 2016, *Summa Theologica.*

"Saint Francis of Assisi," The Humane Society of the United States, accessed May 1, 2017, http://www.humanesociety.org/about/departments/faith/ francis_files/st_francis_of_assisi.html?credit=blog_post_032113_ id4235?referrer=https://www.google.com/.

Joseph G. Sandman, *Centering Prayer: A Treasure for the Soul,* September 9, 2000, America, accessed January 20, 2017, http://www. americamagazine.org/issue/379/article/centering-prayer.

Elizabeth Scott, "The Benefits of Optimism," Very Well, last modified April 28, 2016, accessed December 10, 2016, https://www.verywell.com/the-benefits-of-optimism-3144811.

———, "Types of Stress and Stress Relief Techniques for Each," Very Well, last modified December 31, 2016, accessed December 8, 2016, www. verywell.com/types-of-stress-and-stress-relief-techniques-3144482.

———, "Use Spirituality for Stress Relief," Very Well, last updated July 13, 2016, accessed December 9, 2016, https://www.verywell.com/use-spirituality-for-stress-relief-3144819.

Michael A. Singer, *The Untethered Soul: the journey beyond yourself.* (Oakland: New Harbinger Publications, Inc., 2007).

"Stress in America," America Psychological Association, accessed December 12, 2017, https://www.apa.org/news/press/releases/stress/2010/ national-report.pdf.

"Stress Symptoms, Signs, and Causes," HelpGuide.org, accessed December 8, 2016, https://www.helpguide.org/articles/stress/stress-symptoms-causes-and-effects.htm.

Maryam Taheri, "How to Deal with Stress," Creative Market Blog, accessed December 8, 2016, https://creativemarket.com/blog/how-to-deal-with-stress.

Teresa of Ávila, *The Way of Perfection,* translated and edited by E. Allison Peers, (London: Doubleday, 1946).

"Saint Teresa of Avila Quotes," Brainy Quote, accessed January 28, 2017, www.brainyquote.com/quotes/quotes/s/saintteres586987.html.

"Saint Teresa's Bookmark," *Our Catholic Prayers,* accessed January 30, 2017, http://www.ourcatholicprayers.com/st-teresas-bookmark.html.

Trinity: The Soul of Creation, with Richard Rohr, Cynthia Bourgeault, and Wm Paul Young, Session 2 (April 6-8, 2017). http://cac.org/trinity-webcast/.

Ann and Barry Ulanov, *Primary Speech: A psychology of prayer,* (Atlanta: John Knox Press, 1982).

———, *Religion and the Unconscious,* (Philadelphia: Westminster Press, 1975).

"What is Rigpa," Rigpa, accessed January 28, 2017, http://usa.rigpa.org/about/#_rigpa.

"What is Stress," Explorable, accessed March 5, 2017, https://explorable.com/what-is-stress.

Wendell Berry. *Entries, "To My Mother,"* (Washington: Pantheon Books, 1994).

William Wordsworth, "Surprised by Joy," Poetry Foundation, accessed March 16, 2017, https://www.poetryfoundation.org/poems-and-poets/poems/detail/50285.

John Wright, S.J., *"Prayer," The* New Dictionary of Catholic Spirituality, ed. Michael Downey, (Collegeville: The Liturgical Press, 1993).

Benedict Zimmerman, *"St. John of the Cross," New Advent,* accessed January 18, 2017, http://www.newadvent.org/cathen/08480a.htm.

About the Author

A Catholic priest since 1970, Amato has served more than 20 years as a pastor. He is a graduate of the Shalem Institute in Washington, where he served as adjunct faculty member and is also an Associate of Mepkin Trappist Abbey in South Carolina leading contemplative retreats there. Over the years, he has served on the Spiritual Formation staff of Saint Luke Institute in Maryland and is the co-creator of the Mepkin Priest Wellness Program. He has studied in Rome and Jerusalem. His full-time ministry includes leading days of recollection, retreats, and parish missions. He has Masters degrees in Counseling and in Theology, and a Doctorate in Educational Administration. His prior work on spirituality is *Living in God: Contemplative Prayer and Contemplative Action* published by WestBow Press, 2016.